TUBERCULOSIS: INDIA'S TICKING TIME BOMB

The TB Survivors' Manifesto

TUBERCULOSIS
INDIA'S TICKING TIME BOMB

The TB Survivors' Manifesto

Edited by **CHAPAL MEHRA**

Introduction by **DR SOUMYA SWAMINATHAN,**
Deputy Director General For Programmes, WHO

SPEAKING TIGER

SURVIVORS Against TB

SPEAKING TIGER PUBLISHING PVT. LTD
4381/4, Ansari Road, Daryaganj,
New Delhi—110002, India

First published in India by Speaking Tiger 2018

ISBN: 978-93-87693-18-0
eISBN: 978-93-87693-19-7

Typeset in Sabon by Ram Das Lal, New Delhi
Printed at Shree Maitrey Printech Pvt. Ltd., Noida

CONTENTS

INTRODUCTION: READING AND UNDERSTANDING THIS PATIENT MANIFESTO

There is no interest greater than that of the patients in any healthcare system. If a health system does not recognize and fulfil the patients' needs and safeguard their interests, it is failing in its duty and is unlikely to be a success. This is a fact borne out by numerous health systems and disease control programmes across the world.

If we wish to address and end tuberculosis in India, we must begin by focusing on the common interests of all affected by TB—individuals, families, community and society as a whole. All our efforts must focus on benefitting them, easing their experiences and reducing their suffering.

What are their interests? The best way to understand this is by listening to them. Hence, this critically important survivors' manifesto.

After three decades of diagnosing and treating those affected by TB, I write this introductory note to *Tuberculosis—India's Ticking Time Bomb: The Survivors' Manifesto* with a deep awareness of the failures and successes in the fight against TB in India. We have had numerous successes: the rapid scaling-up of diagnosis and treatment; a robust programme which serves millions and has saved tens of thousands of lives; and an efficient and effectively run system.

Perhaps our greatest shortcoming has been the dearth in understanding the patient experience of fighting and surviving TB. Too easily, we assume their needs, their challenges and their expectations. We convince ourselves of what they need without actually listening to them. We have, at times, been guilty of over-medicalizing this disease, as doctors and public health folks often do. We have often forgotten to see it as a human crisis, a gendered crisis, an economic challenge, and a social and environmental one as well.

Why does this volume matter? It tries to break through these perceptions and requests us to listen to the voices, thoughts and needs of those that have survived TB.

For the first time, patients have identified issues that are relevant to them, as well as discussing an analytical framework around those issues. Until now, patients have been limited to being merely the recipients of care. Rarely have we engaged in thinking through, imagining and designing the care they need and want. This volume departs from that historical approach, and sets forth a new and unambiguous agenda—one where patients take centre stage, identify problems and seek redressal. They suggest solutions that can be implemented by the state but also by the private sector—a vital stakeholder in the fight against TB.

Another key intervention by the patients in this volume is the identification of the set of issues. While including the usual requirements of accurate diagnosis and appropriate treatment, it moves deftly into exploring the social determinants of health, explaining and anyalyzing the critical issues of poverty, hunger, food security, stigma and their impact on TB infection control, diagnosis and treatment. It also explores the crucial area of health communication. These are critically important issues that must be prioritized in the context of patient-centric care.

The structure of this book is unique. Each chapter addresses a different aspect of tackling TB in India. It begins with the author's own story of battling TB and links it to the focus area. The author then explores the issue and provides contextual analysis, for the first time exploring what these challenges mean from a patient perspective. Finally, each chapter and the volume itself ends with a set of recommendations—a patient manifesto, no less—for the health system and all its stakeholders.

India and many other countries have signed up to the World Health Organisation's End TB Strategy, which aims to eliminate TB as a public health problem globally by 2035. While complete elimination may be unachievable, what is important is that every single stakeholder is engaged and working to remove the disease from India. Yet, making TB history will never be possible until we create our plans and strategies on the lines of what those affected by TB expect from us.

Along with the accounts of individual challenges and specific aspects of the fight against TB, this volume provides us with several reminders of the magnitude and depth of India's TB crisis. TB is a curable disease that nevertheless kills thousands of Indians every day. We have startling statistics on the extent of death and suffering left in its wake. The rising tide of drug resistance also threatens to undo the enormous progress India has made in stemming the spread of TB. While TB can affect people of any class, religion, ethnicity and socioeconomic status, it disproportionately affects the most marginalized in society, including children, the homeless, prisoners and people living with HIV/AIDS. The disease has gone beyond being a health crisis alone—it is an economic crisis which costs India close to Rs 15.6 lakh crores (US$ 24 billion) each year and pushes families and communities into debt, and poverty.

I believe efforts like this volume and numerous other recent developments—the commitment by India's political leadership to eliminating TB; the ambitious national strategic plan 2017–2025; and the fact that you now hear and see TB survivors speaking at programmes and events much more frequently—give reason for much hope. The recent decision to provide direct economic benefits to TB patients is perhaps the single most transformative move for TB affected families and individuals.

I urge each and every stakeholder connected with TB to read this volume. Not because the articles are definitive or reflect every aspect of our fight against TB. On the contrary, they articulate the most important and missing aspect of our work with TB—what patients think, and what they need from us, as healthcare providers. It is more than a patient manifesto. It is a call to action against TB. One which we cannot ignore anymore.

Dr Soumya Swaminathan,
Deputy Director General for Programmes,
World Health Organisation (WHO)

EDITOR'S NOTE: UNDERSTANDING TUBERCULOSIS IN INDIA

Chapal Mehra

Termed a ticking time bomb, tuberculosis remains one of India's most significant health challenges, killing over a thousand Indians every day. A curable disease, a stigmatized one, an engine of poverty and debt—TB has numerous manifestations, each of which create difficult circumstances for the individuals, families and communities affected by it.

Despite extensive efforts to control it, TB in India remains elusive, insufficiently understood and ever growing—an untameable epidemic. Although at the highest levels of decision-making, India has committed to eliminating TB, yet we remain unable to conceive its end in the foreseeable future.

Claims of ending TB, well-intentioned and sincere, remain empty while millions grapple with this disease. These claims are also at odds with India's full-blown epidemic of TB and drug-resistant (DR) TB—a crisis that has been decades in the making, due to policies of benign neglect on the part of successive administrations. TB is a staggering epidemic that affects 2.8 million people, pushing individuals, families and communities into poverty, suffering and debt. Such claims then must be borne out by thoughtful strategy and serious commitment, backed by sufficient funding. However, these seem to be missing.

India has a strategic five-year plan to control TB which aims to find, treat, prevent and build for TB control on a massive scale. However, the plan ignores the fact that most Indians affected by TB do not seek care under the government health programme. It is usually their last choice. Even the poorest prefer to pay and go to the private sector because it is efficient and accessible. They land up in the public sector only later, often penniless and much sicker. That most TB-affected people need efficient care with dignity and respect has escaped India's health programme planners.

Combine these concerns with a more dangerous and harder-to-treat drug-resistant form of TB, and the crisis becomes severe—and alarming. A decade of neglect has now resulted in an epidemic of multi-drug-resistant (MDR) TB. India has close to 100,000 cases of MDR TB—many consider this figure to be an underestimation. MDR TB is harder— and also prohibitively expensive—to diagnose and treat. A single case of MDR TB can infect another ten to twenty cases a year, unless the patient is started promptly on effective treatment. In many of India's urban centres, the MDR TB case burden is significant, with some strains resistant to all available drugs, as was reported at Hinduja Hospital in 2012.

These contradictions stem from our limited understanding of what TB is—an ancient disease that can spread through the air and which consumes the patient if not diagnosed and treated early. TB, however, is a lot more than just that in contemporary India. It is not a unidimensional disease but many ailments combined, well beyond its physiological manifestation. Apart from the bacteria, and the physical damage it inflicts, there are deep economic, social and cultural dimensions of TB that remain largely ignored and unaddressed.

Unfortunately, most of the discourse around TB in India emanating from government, the private sector, international partners and the like remains mired in a single approach—test, treat, adhere to the treatment. In truth, those that treat TB and those tasked to manage this epidemic, remain unengaged in what it means to be affected, what the process of fighting TB means to those affected, their families and their community.

This lack of understanding is not deliberate on an individual level. It is a result of following a dominant medical paradigm to address and manage TB for many years. Within this paradigm, even the language used by stakeholders remains that of 'control', 'adherence' and 'education'. There is seldom discussion on understanding the perspectives of those affected—the patients.

Why is TB misunderstood? Perhaps because several of its dimensions are beyond the capacity of the health establishment. A lack of preventive strategies, the prevalence of poor nutrition, and increasingly rapid urbanization, combined with limited public awareness, all feed India's epidemic. These are domains traditionally outside of disease control programmes, though they have an undeniable impact on disease control. In truth, the health establishment is often powerless, despite its sincerest intentions to control this epidemic.

Finding Truth through Representation

If we are to address India's TB problem comprehensively, we must turn to the popular or mainstream understanding of TB. The representation of TB, or consumption as it was once termed, has been romanticized in the West and often depicted poetically. In India, however, this condition has remained associated with poverty, poor hygiene and poor nutrition. Despite being a current and modern crisis, TB has remained a whispered disease, its survivors forced to live in silence—denying them the ability to even talk about their relentless and unforgiving condition while it consumes them.

The popular imagination of TB has not changed much. Even today, a TB patient is treated with fear, trepidation and concern, whether by his/her community, or even in healthcare settings. Discrimination is rampant and treatment is often inhumane. While the disease has changed and evolved, our understanding of it has remained mired in incorrect, often misguided notions. A strange silence persists around TB, our poor understanding of it and our inability as a nation to recognize symptoms and seek care without fear and discrimination. This is at the heart of India's TB crisis.

Perhaps what is most ironic then, is that while public awareness campaigns push those affected by TB to seek care, the stigma around TB pushes them into silence, not merely socially, but in terms of vocally interacting with healthcare professionals and the system. TB treatment and diagnosis can take time. Yet, if a disease requires a long duration of adherence to drugs and management of side effects, then how can the role of the affected individual or community be so diminished? Why do the TB affected have so little say in how the disease is managed, how heathcare systems are structured, and what research priorities are?

While patients can expect very little from the system, the system expects patients to comply entirely—take medicine without lapses, manage side effects, address mental health issues—and entirely on their own. Apart from this, it does little to address their economic, social and individual needs or aspirations. The role of patients is to follow instructions.

Not surprisingly, the TB patient is most often disengaged, and distant from the system and, during treatment, from society at large. Even when cured, most patients are told to bury their experience with TB in the past, like an unpleasant nightmare which they should neither speak of nor discuss with others. Thus, the shame associated with TB continues well after TB is cured. This inability to talk about the disease causes not only silence around TB, but an internalization of the suffering and stigma. Not surprisingly, as a result, TB has few champions or survivors, and even fewer to ask for change or challenge the system.

The TB Patient as Storyteller

The most critical character in the TB story is not the doctor, or the health system, but the patient. While TB affects millions of Indians, very few of them have a say in how they are diagnosed, how they are treated, what information they get, what support they need to defeat this disease, and how to get it. In essence, the character at the epicentre of this journey has no voice.

While working with and listening to the TB affected, or recording their stories, I have found these patients filled with questions—and also with answers. However, they remain disengaged from the health system tasked to address their needs. This is due to multiple reasons, which include fundamental issues such as class, geographical location, ability to access health care, gender and, most critically, stigma. As a result, the narrative of the health system is filled with gaps and inconsistencies. Through this volume and the stories recorded by us, we hope to address some of these gaps and numerous oversights.

The journey of the TB affected is deeply instructive when examined closely. From what makes them vulnerable to why they often abandon treatment, the logic in their narratives is unquestionable. Their ability to negotiate the disease is often limited and their support systems, both within the healthcare system and within their homes, are fragile. Their stories are compelling insights into what it takes to navigate the experience of fighting TB. Hence, the TB survivors themselves became our primary storyteller.

In this book, they recall their stories with support from editors and writers to reconstruct a narrative of their journey. This is critical because patients rarely take centre-stage in telling the TB story from their own perspective. Even when patients do speak, their stories are divided into sound bytes to fit into news articles and policy papers for analysis or momentary shock. In many ways, patients are the visible but voiceless stakeholders of TB—seen but rarely heard. This volume seeks to break that mould.

Why This Volume?

This volume was conceptualized as a patient manifesto and developed to articulate and bring the patient perspective on TB in India to the mainstream. While a significant amount of literature exists on diagnosing and treating TB, little or no documentation exists of how patients experience all the disease stages and what they need to fight TB successfully.

From the time a patient first coughs or finds other signs of TB, to when they take their last dose, patients are expected to follow rules and meet the expectations set by others. The system does not allow for challenge or redressal. The patients' dependence on the system is absolute and their agency limited. Their needs, perspective and demands (if any) remain unarticulated. Through this volume, we are hope to highlight some of these challenges and perspectives and change mindsets.

Sitting in his one-room house in Dharavi, on a rainy Mumbai morning, Owais, India's first patient to be put on Bedaquiline, one of the newest drugs in the arms race against DR TB, once asked me, 'Who would have been responsible if I didn't receive this drug?' In this one question, he sought the answer that most of the TB-affected in India want to know: Do their lives matter? And who is accountable?

When one examines the number of unnecessary TB deaths, the answer may seem apparent. This volume seeks to take that this question further and intends both to be an articulation of demands and to create a process of seeking accountability.

The process of putting it together has been long, requiring extensive work with survivors, interviews with current patients, and with experts. A few key points about the process should also be kept in mind while reading.

Identification of Issues: Several patients and their families, as well as survivors of TB were interviewed before we determined the final list of issues to be discussed in the volume. The notable exceptions to this process were the topics of prevention, urbanization and TB, and research and accountability.

Research and Concept Construction: A team worked with the survivors to help them research and write these chapters. Our goal was to keep their voices strong and authentic, while making the narrative relevant and focussed. In the end, the writing has been done jointly.

Review: Each chapter was reviewed by a leading expert in the field. We worked to incorporate all their suggestions and changes to ensure that the chapters meet the standards of quality and relevance.

At the beginning of each chapter, our focus was to narrate a story and contextualize the analysis and suggestions that followed. Addressing the specific aspect of the disease discussed in the chapter and describing the suffering was critical, as we wanted the narrator to be visible and forthright about their experience and about how the particular issue affected them. The narrator is not just the subject of the narration but also the voice that contextualizes and analyzes the experience, presenting an alternative point of view.

The demands come in a diversity of areas from diagnosis and treatment to empowering TB affected communities and building awareness. There are omissions—research support for TB, and prevention, amongst others. While these are mentioned and discussed, it was not possible to accommodate every issue comprehensively in this volume.

The focus on accountability is both necessary and urgent. India's poorest and most vulnerable have few options—if they go to the public health system they are faced with endless waiting, mistreatment, poor diagnostics and frequent drug shortages. In the private sector, there is poor quality of care and the cost of diagnosing and treating TB is prohibitive, pushing families into debt and poverty. In the end, many give up and disappear, becoming one of the missing million TB patients in India.

Moving Forward

If India wants to address its TB epidemic effectively, it must begin by hearing the voices of survivors and directly affected communities.

It essential that India begin by providing free and accurate diagnosis to every single patient, whether in the public or the private sector. The government also needs to provide all TB patients with an immediate Drug Susceptibility Test (DST), to rapidly identify MDR and more severe forms of DR TB. Instead of giving a standardized regimen, we need to individualize treatment regimens, choosing only drugs which we know the TB bacteria to be sensitive to. The government must also consider introducing, under controlled conditions, new drugs that have the potential for curing the most resistant TB strains.

Simultaneously, we must focus on issues of prevention, community engagement and empowerment. This can be through comprehensive multi-media campaigns to ensure awareness of TB, or community engagement and empowerment programmes to help fight stigma.

Most critically, the government must give up its ambivalence and actively and effectively engage the private sector. That is where India's real crisis of TB exists. TB in India will never be controlled without participation from the private sector. We must learn from experiments currently underway in India where local city governments have transformed how TB is diagnosed and treated, addressing the crisis upfront.

Finally, the programme must recognize the economic and social dimensions of TB. TB often afflicts those between the ages of fifteen to forty-four, leading to poverty and a loss in income. The government has decided to provide Rs 500 for nutritional support to TB patients, but when will this be rolled out? More fundamentally, is this even adequate? We need larger nutritional support programmes and economic support programmes for TB patients and their families during the treatment period, to avoid further impoverishment.

Yet none of this will be possible until sufficient political attention and resources are combined with innovative thinking and a deep focus on the patient to address this imminent crisis. It is instructive to note that India's spending per TB patient is the least among the BRICS countries. The answers lie in expanding the capacity of the public sector, aggressively engaging the private sector, increasing budgets, and creating a massive campaign to ensure awareness and empowerment among those most severely affected. We need access to a free and reliable TB test, counselling, free high-quality treatment, and economic and nutritional support. Until then, TB will continue to devastate the foundations of this aspirational superpower.

DRUG RESISTANT TB: A CRISIS WHICH CAN DESTROY INDIA

Deepti Chavan

My Story: Who am I and why do I write?[1]

I was sixteen years old in 1999, when I first started coughing. I went to our family general practitioner, who prescribed cough medicines. They helped and I got through my exams, yet the cough never really stopped. Finally, a month later, my doctor advised me to get a chest x-ray. I was diagnosed with TB.

After that, although I started taking medication, I remained unwell. We went to one chest physician after another who prescribed one medicine after the next. Nothing helped and my condition continued to worsen.

While I was diagnosed with TB early on, recognizing that it was a drug resistant form took time. My doctor kept changing the medications but never advised me to take a drug-susceptibility test. Most doctors don't suspect drug resistance and hence don't ask patients to get the test done.

After a few months, my doctor at the time told me that part of my left lung had decayed and hence that I required surgery. He also told my parents that I had multi drug-resistant TB. My parents were shocked and worried. We didn't know anything about MDR TB.

I had the recommended surgery in 2000, hoping I would be cured afterwards. I thought I would have to take medicines for few months more, and it will eventually go

---

1 All stories have been prepared by the authors with support and input from their medical providers.

away. I was wrong. After the surgery, I had to continue with the medicines and injections.

Eventually I went to Dr Zarir Udwadia at Hinduja and started treatment with him. I had to give up my place in the engineering course I was attending. After another surgery, which no one thought I'd survive, and many more months of medication, I was finally cured.

I took treatment for MDR TB for six years, during which I took about 400 injections. The medicines had severe side effects: my vision and hearing were affected and I had nausea and joint pains all the time. The worst side effect was from a drug that is basically a dye—my skin became dark. I looked like a skeleton from the weight loss, and seeing myself in a mirror was a nightmare.

Patients affected with MDR TB know so very little about it. Doctors rarely suspect it. Patients are never asked to take a DST. In numerous cases, the degree of resistance is exacerbated due to incorrect treatment. MDR TB is nothing short of a death sentence for thousands of Indians.

I genuinely hope that the government reads this piece and acts to address MDR TB in India!

Drug Resistant TB in India: A crisis decades in the making

DR TB is India's ticking time bomb[2]—a crisis within a crisis. For the uninitiated, it is a strain of TB where the infected person will not respond to, and is resistant to, at least one of the leading TB drugs.[3] There are differing kinds of drug resistance, ranging from MDR TB to

2 Zarir Udwadia refers to TB using this terminology in his landmark TED Talk on TB (available at https://www.youtube.com/watch?v=ziB_OwLda-g). India's staggering TB statistics and rising numbers of DR TB justify this.

3 www.tbfacts.org

extreme (XXDR) and total drug resistance (TDR). The spread of drug resistance is a significant challenge as TB is an air-borne disease, and hence, people can contract the drug resistant strains of the bacteria, each of which are successively more dangerous and complicated to treat.

TB is curable, but recovery from DR TB depends on the kind of resistance, how quickly one is diagnosed and appropriate treatment. The survival rate for MDR TB remains a mere 40 percent globally.[4]

Untreated DR TB has been a holocaust brewing in our own backyard. India is estimated to have 100,000 DR TB cases.[5] This fact became prominent only in 2012 when TDR or XXDR TB cases were reported in Mumbai,[6] leading to a national and international focus on TB. While the government rushed to announce measures, not enough has changed even six years later.

A recent publication in *The Lancet*[7] predicts that by 2040, one in every ten cases in India will be drug resistant, raising the current number of DR TB cases significantly. While numerous concerns have been raised about this study, this news is extremely worrying for India's TB

---

4 WHO data available at http://www.who.int/tb/areas-of-work/drug-resistant-tb/totally-drug-resistant-tb-faq/en/

5 'Multidrug and Extensively Drug Resistant TB (M/XDR TB)', 2010 Global Report on Surveillance and Response, World Health Organisation (WHO). Available at: http://apps.who.int/iris/bitstream/10665/44286/1/9789241599191_eng.pdf

6 Refer to several articles on the emergence of TDR TB, particularly https://www.nature.com/news/totally-drug-resistant-tb-emerges-in-india-1.9797 and http://www.thelancet.com/journals/lancet/article/PIIS0140-6736(12)60085-3/fulltext

7 Mariandyshev, et al, 'Drug Resistant Tuberculosis threatens WHO's End TB Strategy', *The Lancet*, 2017. Available at: http://www.thelancet.com/journals/laninf/article/PIIS1473-3099(17)30246-3/fulltext

control efforts. DR TB remains hard to diagnose and extremely expensive to treat. Thousands of cases of DR TB remain undiagnosed and hence untreated, infecting numerous others.

Many in the government establishment dismiss these fears as alarmist. As an MDR TB survivor, I can tell you MDR TB is a nightmare. Even today, DR TB patients in India can take as long as a year to access correct treatment, largely due to the delays in access to timely and rapid diagnostic molecular technologies that are either too expensive or unfamiliar to most private healthcare providers. The result—human suffering, rising costs and increased transmission.

Why is DR TB a Crisis for India's TB Patients?

When we speak from the patient perspective of challenges that need to be overcome to address India's DR TB crisis, we see a multi-dimensional problem. These factors include:

Poor awareness among health professionals:[8] Despite all the press and awareness efforts, DR TB is rarely suspected by doctors and a DST is often ordered too late. Doctors both in the public and private sectors display poor awareness of the disease leading to rising costs, patient suffering and, in some cases, amplifying resistance through incorrect treatment.

---

8 While there isn't enough data on this issue, we can refer to the anecdotal evidence collected by Survivors Against TB via numerous patient stories. Also refer to Udwadia's work on TB generally. Udwadia et al, 'Tuberculosis Management by Private Practitioners in Mumbai, India: Has Anything Changed in Two Decades?', *NCBI,* 2010. Available at: https://www.ncbi.nlm.nih.gov/pmc/articles/PMC2918510/ We can extrapolate from this to ascertain the poor level of awareness among medical practitioners about DR TB.

Inaccessible diagnoses: DR TB is often diagnosed late in both the public and private sectors. In the public system, rapid diagnostic technologies available at the field level are not used optimally, whereas in the private sector, these tests remain prohibitively expensive and inaccessible. Recently, there were reports of shortages in the cartridges needed for these machines. What's worse is that most Indians who seek care in the private sector cannot access the tests, due to their cost. The rationale for this barrier to access is unclear, because after all, the tests are already funded by public money and ideally should be readily available to all patients. The insufficient use of these technologies leads to overlooking primary drug resistance in patients and therefore, the wrong treatment.

Difficult, expensive and often incorrect treatment: Even if DR TB is diagnosed correctly, taking treatment for it poses severe challenges. In the private sector, most patients cannot afford the Rs 2.5–3 lakhs[9] that such treatment costs. In the public sector, individualized treatment continues to be widely unavailable.[10] All this adds to patient suffering and reduces the ability to fight DR TB.

Some patients can suffer severe side effects, making treatment unmanageable. The treatment itself is of long duration, taking one-and-a-half to two years. These factors add up, and completing treatment for DR TB requires family support, guidance, good counselling, close

---

9 Udwadia et al, 'The Health Economics of Treating MDR TB in Indian Private Sector', *European Respiratory Journal*, 2016. Available at: http://erj.ersjournals.com/content/48/suppl_60/PA1536

10 Udwadia et al, 'Tuberculosis Management by Private Practitioners in Mumbai, India: Has Anything Changed in Two Decades?', *NCBI*, 2010. Available at: https://www.ncbi.nlm.nih.gov/pmc/articles/PMC2918510/

laboratory monitoring and money—almost all of which are missing in both private and public sectors.

Increasing rates of transmission: Excessive delays in providing correct treatment to patients allow networks of disease transmission to be created. The primary prevention of transmission through stringent infection control measures, in both healthcare settings and community life, does not take priority in control measures.[11] If transmission remains ill-understood and continues to be unabated, the cumulative components of TB control will be reduced to a fire-fighting exercise.[12]

There are numerous other challenges as well, such as stigma and poverty, which are addressed in separate chapters. These remain the most significant from the point of view of patients.

What Was Promised?

Over two National Strategic Plans (NSPs), and through speeches made by health ministers, the government has made numerous commitments for addressing MDR TB. These include:

- *Universal DST for TB patients*: However, this is feebly implemented: most patients do not get access to DST easily in the public sector, and in the private sector, patients cannot access the tests for free.

---

11 While there is reference to contact tracing etc. in the NSP, we see very little of this being implemented. We also need work on increased infection control which is currently missing.

12 Mariandyshev et al, 'Drug Resistant Tuberculosis threatens WHO's End TB Strategy', *The Lancet*, 2017. Available at: http://www.thelancet.com/journals/laninf/article/PIIS1473-3099(17)30246-3/fulltext

- *Universal access to DR TB treatment*: This has remained rhetorical because patients in the private sector still cannot access DR TB treatment easily in the public sector.

What Do Patients Need?

If India is serious about addressing DR TB, these are key suggestions from the survivor perspective to ensure a comprehensive redressal.

India needs to start by being honest. The country announced a DR TB survey three years ago, which has released no numbers till date. Why are the results not available? We need to understand truly how large the epidemic is to plan for the quantum of technologies and drugs we require to fight DR TB. Secondly, there is no continuous surveillance—despite TB being a notifiable disease, not every provider informs government authorities of TB cases—and the building of a health management information system though data from molecular diagnostics is woefully absent. **We need to count every DR TB case irrespective of where they seek care.**

A large section of India seeks care for DR TB in the private sector. The government must create an effective partnership which ensures that every DR TB case is diagnosed and treated efficiently without unnecessary costs or delays. The ethical responsibility of ensuring this lies with the government which is tasked with disease control. India cannot address its DR TB crisis until all patients are given the same free diagnosis and treatment. **Everyone must have access to free and accurate diagnosis and treatment.**

How do communities and people address and recognize DR TB? We need large-scale awareness in providers and patients. Awareness remains very poor and as a result DR TB is diagnosed late and often treated inappropriately.

We also urgently need prevention programmes that can help those at risk. These come from recognizing TB symptoms early, creating awareness among all populations and the medical community, and renewing focus on the fundamentals of disease prevention, nutrition, improved housing, income security and access to health services. **Every Indian needs to know and understand the dangers and symptoms of TB.**

India must enhance its laboratory capacity and provide every TB patient with up-front drug susceptibility testing, to rapidly identify all forms of DR TB. Even though a vast number of machines to diagnose DR TB are available, the tests in India's public sector remain rationed. **Every Indian should have access to free, reliable diagnosis for DR TB as and when required.**

India must ensure access to free and high-quality treatment for DR TB patients irrespective of where they seek care. It must provide access to the two new drugs, Bedaqualine and Delamanid, particularly to patients in the private sector. This remains limited as a recent case illustrated.[13] **No Indian should be denied new drugs irrespective of where they seek care.**

Patients and families affected by DR TB suffer stress and information gaps and require counselling. India needs to create a patient support system which includes counselling, nutritional and economic support. **We must provide every Indian not just treatment but the support they need for fighting TB.**

Finally, India must ensure that DR TB does not lead families into debt and poverty. This should address all TB patients and not just those who seek care in the

---

13 See Mehra, Chapal. 'How to Kill a TB Patient', Huffington Post, 2017. Available at: http://www.huffingtonpost.in/chapal-mehra/how-to-kill-a-tb-patient_a_21652415/

government system. While economic support has been proposed, its implementation still remains questionable. **We need every patient to be provided economic support through a transparent and accountable system without hurdles such as Aadhar and other barriers to access.**

THE PRIVATE SECTOR AND TB

Saurabh Rane

My Story

I was training to be a doctor when I started feeling sick. After two weeks of continued fever, cough and immense weight loss, we decided to go for an x-ray and found I had fluid in my left lung. The doctor told me that it was TB.

I was started on medication but didn't feel better even after a few months. Given my medical training, I knew something was wrong. I persuaded the doctor to get a drug sensitivity test done. Yet nothing conclusive was found and my treatment continued, based on what, I am not sure. I developed high fever again and lost more weight.

In confusion and exasperation, I pushed my doctor for a left lung sonography to determine the cause of fever. During the sonography, my doctor accidentally moved his hand to my right lung. There were close to 1000 cc of fluid in my right lung. I was devastated, because now both my lungs were infected.

I lost faith in my doctor and went in for a second opinion. My new doctor advised further tests, especially a culture to diagnose my drug resistance. Tests revealed I was a highly drug-resistant case. I could not believe it—especially because I know that the success rate of treatment for cases like mine was barely 20 percent. Also, treatment was long, expensive, and came with multiple side effects. My treatment lasted for over two-and-a-half years—months of extreme side effects, high costs, anxiety and mental fatigue. If it was not for my family and a few friends, I would not have survived this.

TB affects 2.8 million Indians every year. While I sought treatment in the private sector, what we really need is free high-quality diagnosis and treatment irrespective of whether one is diagnosed in the private or public sector.

Anyone can get TB; what is critical is to have access to easy, affordable and quality diagnosis and medicines. Hopefully, policy makers in India will read this piece and make the changes we need to end TB.

TB and the Private Sector

India has one of the world's largest and most diverse private health sectors. From qualified doctors to quacks to 'jhola wala' practitioners—everyone treats everything, simple and complex ailments alike. Despite its heterogeneity, the private sector remains one of the largest providers of health services in the country. According to the National Sample Survey Office (NSSO), over 70 percent of Indians (72 percent in rural India and 79 percent in urban India) seek care in the private sector at one point or another.[14] This poses challenges but also enormous opportunities for ensuring access to affordable, accurate and reliable high-quality treatment and healthcare services.

In the case of TB, the majority of patients initially seek treatment in the private sector, even though the government provides free treatment and diagnosis. There are numerous reasons for this, of which ease of access and perceived quality of care are amongst the leading ones. In urban areas, ease of access, flexible timings and

14 Health India, NSS 71st Round, January–June 2014. Available at: http://mospi.nic.in/sites/default/files/publication_reports/nss_rep574.pdf

behaviour of healthcare staff are considered prominent reasons to avoid public sector facilities. Another associated reason is concern about confidentiality.

At the same time, diagnosis and treatment of TB in India's vast private sector remains of uneven quality and, many argue, can even be an engine of drug resistance. Yet millions prefer the private sector. This poses interesting challenges about balancing patient choice and quality of care in India.

Traditionally, an average TB patient has a long and somewhat schizophrenic trajectory. They often swing between the private and public sectors as funds run out and a final cure remains difficult to obtain. In most cases, there is some interface with the private sector. Clearly, TB in India cannot be ended until the private sector is engaged effectively. This means that the government needs to employ new and innovative strategies to engage and work with the private sector.

What Challenges Does the Private Sector Pose for TB?

From the patient perspective, as well as from the perspective of disease control, the private sector is fraught with numerous challenges. These include but are not limited to the following:

Diagnosis: TB diagnosis can be a challenge, as the private sector prescribes a plethora of tests for TB diagnosis. Many of these tests are inappropriate for TB detection and are riddled with their own unique challenges. For instance, liquid culture testing takes weeks to provide a result. It is costly and can only be carried out by highly trained staff in specialist laboratories. Similarly, the nucleic acid amplification test (NAAT), which is widely recognized as one of the most efficient means of testing TB, has diagnostic cartridges with a short shelf-life, operating temperature and humidity restrictions, requires a continuous electricity supply and needs annual servicing and calibration of each machine.

Treatment: Private providers have poor compliance with the Revised National TB Control Programme (RNTCP)/ World Health Organization (WHO) treatment regimens, with errors in both dosage of drugs and duration of treatment.[15] Also, poor usage of proper adherence methodologies leads to low adherence among patients. Many view this as a genesis for drug resistance in India.

Expense: The costs of diagnosis and treatment remain prohibitive in the private sector. Most patients cannot afford quality care without financial strain. This also makes treatment adherence a challenge. In many cases, patients are forced to stop their course of treatment due to the high costs of medicines, tests or consultations in the private sector. Because of its profit-seeking nature, the private sector also has no system of monitoring to ensure that patients complete treatment.

Uneven quality of care: This is both a function of the heterogeneous nature of private providers, their limited skill levels and its poor understanding of TB. This leads to delayed diagnoses, poor diagnostic and treatment practices, and poor compliance with TB treatment. Further, follow-up care, such as contact tracing, co-infection (diabetes and HIV) screening and prophylaxis, remains feeble. This is a function of the numerous quacks and less-qualified providers in the private sectors who treat and diagnose TB.

---

15 Udwadia, Pinto and Uplekar, 'Tuberculosis Management by Private Practitioners in Mumbai, India: Has Anything Changed in Two Decades?', PLoS One, 2010. Source: http://journals.plos.org/plosone/article?id=10.1371/journal.pone.0012023

Lack of counselling and support: There is virtually no engagement of patients and their families via TB counselling and support. As a result, families do not understand the importance of care for TB-affected individuals, and patients themselves do not receive much needed support for the issues they face during TB treatment. Widespread information and awareness building campaigns for patients and their families are needed. However, these are completely missing in the private sector.

Why is Working Together a Challenge?

From a systemic point of view, there are numerous challenges to the public and private sector working together.

The private sector complains about the absence of information and outreach from the public sector TB programme.[16] The constant refrain is that the government doesn't do much to engage them.

Being profit-led, the private sector finds itself unable to respond to government schemes with limited incentives and is more focussed on numbers. Private practitioners admit that they may be unable to take on certain tasks, such as tracing those who miss taking medicines, providing social support to patients, and detailed record keeping and analysis.

There is a lack of resolve in the public sector to address the challenges in the private sector.[17] National TB Programme

---

16 Ibid.

17 Uplekar et al, 'Private Practitioners and Public Health: Weak Links in Tuberculosis Control', *The Lancet*, vol 358, issue 9285, 2001, pp. 912–16, http://www.thelancet.com/journals/lancet/article/PIIS0140-6736(01)06076-7/fulltext?_eventId=login

(NTP)[18] managers do not consider the private sector as a factor. The managers believe that eventually patients will turn away from exploitative and profit-oriented private practitioners. Others perceive the private sector as an unmanageable entity.

In many cases, public sector managers are too preoccupied with the DOTS programmes. They are apprehensive about addressing the additional challenges that the private sector poses.

Other constraints include a lack of willingness, as well as the necessary skills and human resources to work with the private sector. Nonetheless, there is general agreement on the need to act to get private practitioners on board.

What Commitments Have Been Made?

The National Strategic Plan (2012–2017) ensured early and improved diagnosis of all TB patients, improved outreach, expansion of case-finding efforts, and deploying better diagnostic services to patients diagnosed and treated in the private sector.

The recent National Strategic Plan (2017–2025) specifies the provision of free diagnosis and treatment in the private sector. Strategies to control TB through public-sector health services will have little impact if inappropriate management of TB patients in private clinics continues unabated. While little has changed over the years, we are hopeful that the private sector will comply with the latest suggestions in the NSP.

18 Dr Mukund Uplekar employs the term NTP in his comparative analysis of TB control programmes in various countries.

What Do Patients Need from Private and Public Sector Healthcare?

Assured quality of care: It is the patient's choice about where to seek care. Irrespective of where individuals seek care, it is important that the government ensures enforcement and accountability so that healthcare is reliable and affordable. The RNTCP has developed formal guidelines to help local programmes structure collaborations with private healthcare providers and non-governmental organizations. The guidelines need to be enforced stringently. **Every citizen affected by TB should be assured of appropriate diagnosis and treatment in the private sector.**

Seamless access through public–private partnerships: The private sector can play a pivotal role in controlling TB in India. In the interest of disease control, we need to collaborate with the private sector. This will help outreach in hard-to-reach areas, including remote rural areas. It will also lead to increased case detection and notification of TB cases.[19] A strong system of referrals from the private to the public sector will scale up diagnostic and treatment services for TB and DR TB.[20] **In the end, every TB affected individual should have seamless access to care either through the public or private sectors.**

---

19 Bhatia, Vineet, 'Enhancing Private Sector Contribution to TB Care in India', *Samm Health International*, 2010, page 14, http://www.tbpartnershipindia.org/documents/Enhancing%20private%20sector%20contribution%20to%20TB%20care%20in%20India.pdf

20 Uplekar et al, 'Private Practitioners and Public Health: Weak Links in Tuberculosis Control', *The Lancet,* Vol 358, Issue 9285, 2001, pp. 912–916, http://www.thelancet.com/journals/lancet/article/PIIS0140-6736(01)06076-7/fulltext?_eventId=login

Free and affordable care: The government aims to provide universal access to quality diagnosis and treatment to end TB by 2025. However, even today most private sector patients do not have access to free diagnosis and treatment without enrolling in the government programme. **Every patient must be able to access free diagnosis and treatment in the private sector.** This can be done easily by following options in partnership with the private sector:

- Participation in referring, diagnosing and treating patients with TB;
- Establishing TB treatment centres within a private healthcare facility and
- Conducting training and workshops with private laboratories.[21]

Counselling: The government needs to ensure that every patient receives appropriate counselling through the government as well as the private sector, empowering them with sufficient information to deal with the disease and also providing the appropriate support systems to manage the disease. **Every TB affected family must be provided appropriate counselling and information in their regional language both in the public and private sectors.** The government needs to establish protocols for this.

Involve key stakeholders: Other suggestions include reviewing the current approaches to engaging the private sector in TB care and control, and redesigning these through consultations with key stakeholders, including healthcare professionals, NGOs, the pharmaceutical industry, etc.[22]

---

21 Dewan, P. 'Improving Tuberculosis Control through Public–Private Collaboration in India: Literature Review', *BMJ* 2006, 332, 574, http://www.bmj.com/content/332/7541/574

22 Udwadia, Pinto and Uplekar (2010) 'Tuberculosis Management

The Government of India has rolled out a direct benefit transfer scheme for patients on TB treatment. This is a huge step in the right direction which will help TB patients complete their treatment and recover completely. However, the implementation of this scheme needs to be effective and translate on the ground. Similarly, information and communication technology-based portals such as NIKSHAY[23] need to become broad-based and reach the grassroots for effective TB prevention and control. The government is also in the process of rolling out 99 DOTS, which offers a fixed-dose combination of TB medicines. This is another welcome step, although its implementation has been slow.

India needs to urgently address its private sector challenge if it wants to end TB by 2025. In the end, this will not be possible until every Indian has access to free, accurate and patient-centric care in both the public and the private sector.

---

by Private Practitioners in Mumbai, India: Has Anything Changed in Two Decades?' PLoS ONE 5(8): e12023. doi:10.1371/journal.pone.0012023

23 To monitor the RNTCP effectively, a web-enabled and case-based monitoring application called NIKSHAY has been developed by the National Informatics Centre. This is used by health functionaries at various levels across the country in association with the Central TB Division and the Ministry of Health & Family Welfare. NIKSHAY covers various aspects of addressing TB using technological innovations. Apart from web-based technology, SMS-services have been used effectively for communication with patients and monitoring the programme on day-to-day basis. See: https://nikshay.gov.in/AboutNikshay.htm

DIAGNOSIS: TECHNIQUES AND TACTICS

Debshree Lokhande

My Story

I am an architect who contracted TB six-and-a-half years ago in Ahmadabad. We still have not been able to determine whether it started out as Drug Sensitive TB or its dangerous cousin, MDR TB. When I developed a persistent cough and sudden extreme fever, the doctor suspected a viral infection. He also asked for a chest x-ray. The x-ray gave no exact diagnosis, although the radiologist did make a prophetic statement: 'You're going to be taking medicines for a long time!'

It wasn't long before I moved back to my home town, Pune. We consulted a private chest physician who prescribed the first-line TB drug, Rifampicin, and other second-line drugs. All these drugs were prescribed without testing me for TB. The doctor referred us to a microbiologist who was his friend. The report stated that I was sensitive to Rifampicin as well as Cycloserine. As a result, along with Rifampicin and Cycloserine, I was also prescribed Amikacin and Moxicilin. All strong drugs.

Four weeks and another sputum test later, it was revealed that I had become resistant to Cycloserine as well. While this drug was stopped, the others were continued, including those that the report said I was sensitive to. Amikacin was stopped after two months only, whereas ideally it should be taken for six months.

Fast forward to a year later: I became resistant to Rifampicin and finally this drug too was dropped from my daily cocktail of TB drugs. This is where the resistance pattern changed drastically, following which the doctor altered my prescription—after one whole year. Had we been aware that TB tests are more reliable when conducted by bigger hospitals, who actually follow international guidelines, we would have never visited the doctor's microbiologist friend.

And just like that, incorrect reports, resulting in several changes to treatment within a span of three years, left me weaker and highly drug-resistant. Those three years took a toll on my body, destroying my left lung. I also lost my hearing, which was a side effect of one of the injectable drugs. Had my doctor prescribed a GeneXpert at an early stage, I would have found out earlier that I had become resistant to the first-line drugs.

It was a straightforward conclusion for me. Repeated wrong diagnostic tests and the consequent repeated changes to my treatment regimen worsened my condition. Finally, it was in Mumbai that I was finally put on therapy to salvage the situation. I was approved for Bedaquiline and took it for six months. I improved, I felt better, and also managed to have my hearing restored through cochlear implant technology.

However, a year later, my cough returned with partial weight loss. I was advised a surgery which would completely remove my damaged left lung. After the surgery, I was again put on a course of both Delaminid and Bedaquiline, for a period of six months. And finally, for the first time in six long years, my sputum turned negative.

I am a living example of how the wrong diagnosis can destroy everything: years of my life, much of my social circle, and my entire family's savings. I hope this piece will get the stakeholders to focus on the diagnosis of TB as a critical issue.

The TB Diagnostic Landscape in India

India's healthcare system is divided into the public and private healthcare sectors. The two sectors approach TB diagnosis differently. The challenges both face are accurate testing and early detection of drug resistance.

Public sector: Sputum smear microscopy, the most widely used method of TB diagnosis in the public sector, misses more than half of all cases[24] and is ineffective in patients with HIV–TB co-infection. While, Xpert, a more reliable, though expensive, test, is easily available in urban areas, its availability in the rural areas remains poor and somewhat rationed. More recently though, TrueNaat, which is a new indigenous molecular test, will be brought into use to diagnose TB in an hour, while also indicating whether the patient has resistance to Rifampicin.

Private sector: More than half of India's TB patients are managed through the private sector,[25] where the quality of care is variable. Usually, the private sector prescribes several tests for TB diagnosis. However, these tests are all riddled with their own unique challenges.

Interferon Gamma Release Assays (IGRAs): Globally, IGRAs are used to diagnose Latent TB Infection (LTBI). Latent TB means that the TB bacteria is present in one's body but in a dormant form. Based on WHO guidelines it is clear that IGRAs are not be used for

24 'Why is research essential to stop TB', Stop TB Partnership, www.stoptb.org/global/research/funding.asp

25 National Strategic Plan 2012–2017, Central TB Division, Directorate General of Health Services, Ministry of Health and Family Welfare, p. 30. Available at: https://www.tbfacts.org/wp-content/uploads/2016/01/NSP-2012-2017.pdf

active TB diagnosis.[26] On June 7, 2012 the Government of India banned the use of serology (blood tests) for TB detection. These have however now been replaced by IGRAs in multiple labs. IGRAs are being increasingly misused to diagnose active TB. Such a scenario leads to overtreatment, which is detrimental for the overall health of the population.[27] If that's not enough, one test can cost as much as Rs 2000 to Rs 3000.[28]

Liquid culture testing: The most sensitive test, the liquid culture test takes weeks to provide a result. But this is the gold standard and any drug can be tested for resistance. The isolated mycobacteria can also be subjected to various other tests if required, later on. The test is costly and can only be carried out by highly trained staff in specialist laboratories. This poses the challenge of affordability and limits follow ups.

Nucleic acid amplification technologies (NAAT): These include Xpert MTB/RIF (GeneXpert's academic name: MTB=*Mycobacterium tuberculosis*/Resistant to Rifampicin). They reduce the turnaround time of diagnosing TB and drug resistance to two hours and can be used at decentralized locations. However, NAAT too has its own limitations, including the limited shelf-life of the diagnostic cartridges, operating temperature and humidity restrictions, requiring a continuous electricity

---

26 'Use of Interferon Gamma Release Assays (IGRAs) in low and middle income countries', Policy Statement, World Health organisation (WHO), 2011. Available at: http://apps.who.int/iris/bitstream/10665/44759/1/9789241502672_eng.pdf

27 Little et al, 'Costs and Consequences of using Interferon Gamma Release Assays for the Diagnosis of Active TB in India', PLoS One, 2015. Source: http://journals.plos.org/plosone/article?id=10.1371/journal.pone.0124525

28 Ibid

supply and annual servicing and calibration of each machine. This test also remains prohibitively expensive in the private sector.

Line probe assay (LPA): This test is primarily recommended for first- and second-line drug susceptibility. It is a molecular test and the results take two to five days. In the public sector, this test is offered free of cost.

Increasingly, India has moved towards adopting and scaling up GeneXpert as the preferred mode of TB diagnosis. The Government of India has rolled out GeneXpert across eighteen sites with 400 machines across the country. However, this technique is expensive in the private sector. The public sector on the other hand, has been slow in rolling out GeneXpert across the country.

Why is TB Diagnosis Such a Challenge?

The diagnosis of TB is riddled with severe challenges regardless of which sector a patient approaches. The reasons for them are many:

TB is not even considered for diagnosis when a symptomatic patient visits the doctor with persistent cough. Hence, there is a considerable time lapse between the first visit to the doctor and the actual diagnosis of TB. It is estimated that two to six months are lost in seeking the correct diagnosis,[29] and that an individual with TB can infect ten to fifteen people every year,

---

29 'Time of Action on TB Communication, A briefing for policy makers, programmers and health communicators on contemporary communication opportunities and challenges', Panos Policy Briefing, London, 2005. Available at: http://www.stoptb.org/assets/documents/countries/acsm/Action%20on%20TB%20Communications%20(PANOS).pdf

if not diagnosed and treated on time. **TB remains underdiagnosed in India.**

Even if a person is considered for TB diagnosis, s/he is often subject to wrong diagnostic techniques. For instance, IGRA, which should ideally be used to detect latent TB infection, is being used for active TB diagnosis. Those who are wrongly diagnosed and therefore subjected to unnecessary TB treatment also develop higher chances of becoming drug resistant. **Lack of correct and timely diagnosis** not only perpetuates the cycle of TB transmission, but also results in the TB bacteria turning drug resistant.

With the emergence of DR TB, the importance of conducting **universal drug sensitivity tests** has become even more critical. A DST allows doctors to determine whether a person is drug resistant or not. This is critical in the management of DR TB. It helps in developing a tailor-made treatment regimen for every person infected with TB. Unfortunately, DST is not considered early. As a result, many drug resistant patients end up being misdiagnosed and hence, following wrong treatment regimens. Such a scenario leads to increased drug resistance transmission.

In both sectors there are often **shortages** of relevant cartridges etc. so those seeking diagnostic tests often have to wait or do not have accurate tests available.

Over-the-counter availability of broad spectrum antibiotics like ciprofloaxicin is driving multi-drug resistance at a fast pace. In India, any person can walk to the pharmacist and get few tablets of ciprofloxacon (ciprobid) for any ailment, including the common cold, fever, loose motions, etc. The patient takes a sub-optimal dose for one to two days and after relief of symptoms (which may be spontaneous), stops these drugs. This **indiscriminate availability of antibiotics** is leading to the drugs of this class becoming highly ineffective for any treatment.

Ineffective and inaccurate diagnostics in the public and private sector lead to patient suffering and help spread infection, fuelling India's TB epidemic. The last two NSPs (2012–2017 and 2017–2025), promise universal access to quality diagnosis and treatment. Till date, this has not been implemented effectively. TB is curable if accurately detected and treated in time. Timely and correct diagnosis curtails the cycle of TB transmission and aids in commencing TB treatment at the earliest.

What Can Be Done?

India needs to provide a reliable and accurate TB test to any symptomatic who walks in. **Everyone deserves accurate, free and high quality diagnosis.** There should be no discrimination based on where one seeks treatment and who your doctor is. Engaging with the private sector by providing clear medical guidelines and rationales for compulsory testing will go a long way in curbing the problem of TB.

There needs to be an **accelerated roll out of universal GeneXpert across India in both public and private healthcare sectors.** It needs to be made accessible to all people so that faster diagnosis and hence commencement of treatment is made possible.

All doctors across India must prescribe a DST to all patients diagnosed with TB. This will help in determining the drug resistance status of an individual and improve the treatment offered. **Every Indian diagnosed with TB must have access to DST.**

The government needs to strategize and plan the stocks required for TB tests. A clear forecasting mechanism needs to be put in place to ensure that TB patients in India do not suffer because of lack of drugs. **Shortages should be unacceptable in the public or private sectors.**

Hasten the process of introducing new tests across India. There is a need to study and evaluate the performance of new diagnostic tests on the basis of feasibility, cost-effectiveness, reduced diagnostic delay, impact on clinical decision-making and patient benefit.

Strategic, targeted and informed public information campaigns to increase public awareness will help communities identify the symptoms of TB and seek appropriate care. The campaign must include information on TB, its symptoms and where/how to obtain care, as well as diagnosis.

A greater focus on research and development is needed to develop indigenous diagnostic solutions which are cost-effective, as well as to explore ways to combine existing and new diagnostics for timely and accurate diagnosis of various strains of TB. It is equally critical to monitor and evaluate each of these diagnostic techniques to ensure efficacy and accuracy. Regular assessment and quality control of diagnostic services and upgradation of equipment will ensure that the TB diagnostic industry remains well-funded. **India must invest in making its own tests tailored to addressing its epidemic.**

A patients' grievance cell, hotline or website needs to be in place so that they can they can clarify doubts themselves. Further, a thorough assessment of all microbiologists and technicians in relation to their backgrounds, levels of commitment and honesty is critical to ensure that no patient suffers.

There exists a critical need for **policy interventions** to stringently implement the ban on serology-based tests for TB detection, as well as to ban the use of IGRAs in the private sector for active TB diagnosis.

India cannot address its TB crisis until it ensures universal access to reliable, accurate and free TB diagnosis. DR TB needs to be diagnosed early to reduce costs, human suffering and transmission rates. In the end, we should not forget that timely and accurate diagnosis equals lives saved!

TREATMENT ADHERENCE AND CHALLENGES

Arun Singh

My Story

Seven years ago, my father died of TB. I was a young physiotherapy student then, doing an internship. My family had taken dad to a renowned private hospital in Delhi, where he underwent innumerable tests. He was given medicines based on a vague diagnosis. In the end, it was at a government hospital where he was finally diagnosed with TB. By then however, it was too late and crucial time had been lost.

While I was trying to piece my life together after dad's demise, TB came back to haunt me. I found I was coughing over a few weeks and so I went to a physician who prescribed some medicines. However, my condition only worsened. Finally, an x-ray revealed that the lower lobe of my left lung had collapsed.

I was diagnosed with water in my lung. Since further tests could not determine the cause or come to any concrete conclusion medically, doctors decided to put me on TB treatment. By now, I was working as a public health professional and, given my career choice and prior brush with TB, I was stronger and more confident.

After the intensive treatment phase of the first two months, my doctor wanted to change my treatment to a two-drug regimen. I was not convinced and discussed the changing treatment guidelines for TB with my doctor. But he brushed me aside. I was again reminded how disempowered patients are and how little say they have in their own treatments. I downloaded the WHO-endorsed treatment regimen, which comprises three pills a day. I also called my friends in Central Division of TB (CTD) and confirmed that the TB treatment regimen was indeed being changed. In the end, I managed to get the required treatment.

My training in medicine and public health gave me the ability to understand the treatment protocols and change my treatment. Yet, thousands in India suffer from incorrect treatment for an easily treatable disease. I had family support and education. How do those without support and sufficient knowledge survive side effects, stigma and depression? I had the economic ability to afford and complete a full course of the treatment. What happens to those who don't? I hope this chapter will help all stakeholders understand the challenges patients face with regard to treatment, and create change.

Why is Treatment Adherence a Challenge?

There are several factors which contribute to the lack of complete TB treatment at the patient level. The first and foremost challenge is the toxicity of the treatment. This aspect is specifically true for the drug resistant forms of TB. While side effects manifest differently in different individuals, even the milder side effects can cause massive mental and physical challenges. For instance, some patients may experience nausea, headaches, a burning sensation in palms and soles, skin rashes, pins and needles, joint pains, amongst others. Severer side effects include jaundice, depression, mood swings, loss of hearing and/or sight and overall confusion.

Other risk factors can also interfere with TB treatment. For instance, alcohol consumption exacerbates the condition of TB patients. Coupled with a lack of adequate nutrition, alcoholism is likely to lead to severe reactions including nausea and vomiting. This leads to non-adherence to treatment.[30] Often, there is a lack of information and adequate warning about the side effects, and the knowledge of how to counter them is missing in a patient-provider relationship. Further, the lack of attention to the impact of the side effects by healthcare providers is often cited by patients as one of the reasons for treatment non-adherence. As a result, a TB patient is unable to cope and does not complete the treatment at all, or in time.

The second critical factor that deters a TB patient from completing treatment is the deep-rooted stigma associated with TB. This stigma, which is perpetrated by society even now, pushes a TB patient into hiding. Rampant discrimination at the workplace and in all public spaces forces a patient to either hide their treatment or quit their jobs. Stigma may also make patients afraid to ask for support from their employer to purchase medication, thereby reducing adherence.[31] Additional work-related issues include difficulty in obtaining sick leave for treatment, and fear of losing work or of dismissal.

Further, the stigma of TB takes a deeper toll on women. Given our patriarchal society, there have been instances of women being thrown out of their houses,

---

30 Bagchi, Suparna et al, 'Determinants of Poor Adherence to Anti-tuberculosis Treatment in Mumbai, India', *International Journal of Preventive Medicine*, vol 1, no. 4, page 223, 2010, http://ijpm.mui.ac.ir/index.php/ijpm/article/view/30

31 Munro, Salla et al, 'Patient Adherence to Tuberculosis Treatment: A Systematic Review of Qualitative Research,' PLOS Medicine, http://www.plosmedicine.org/article/info:doi/10.1371/journal.pmed.0040238

being isolated, neglected and left to fend for themselves. TB patients hide their diagnosis, feel guilty and ashamed because of the disease. All these factors have adverse effects on treatment completion.

There is also the challenge of costs associated with TB treatment. The private sector for instance, is a profit-driven entity. Consequently, the costs of TB diagnosis, drugs and treatment are exorbitant. These costs are further compounded by additional out-of-pocket expenditure for travel to qualified facilities and consultancy fees. In public healthcare settings where TB treatment is administered free of cost, hidden costs associated with hospital stays, review of x-ray results and travel are high.

TB particularly affects a large number of India's poor due to social, economic and environmental factors. Of these, poverty and under-nutrition are well-established risk factors for TB. Evidence has shown that both these factors are also directly linked to completing TB treatment and its recovery. People with TB frequently experience severe economic barriers to accessing healthcare, including the high expense of diagnosis and treatment, as well as indirect costs due to loss of income. For example, daily wage earners end up losing a whole day's pay if they need to travel to a healthcare facility for a refill. Due to the latter, TB induced poverty can push families into debt traps affecting treatment adherence and completion.

Lack of treatment completion increases the chances of infection, relapse and even death. This has significant human and economic costs. To put it in context, if a family loses its breadwinner to TB, it not only endures the loss of a loved one but has to face steep financial loses. It is like restarting your life from zero.

Research suggests that a significant factor that contributes to treatment completion and adherence is the relationship between the patient and the healthcare provider.[32] There have been instances of TB patients being shunned by providers. Cases of misbehaviour are rampant: for example, some patients have reported that they have been asked to stand outside in the burning sun, once diagnosed.

Even if the provider doesn't contribute to the stigma, there is hardly any space for a dialogue between a provider and a patient. Yet, a TB patient's rate of treatment success is directly proportional to the patient's relationship with the healthcare provider. Seeking help for TB requires a lot of courage and determination on the part of the patient. However, healthcare providers do not treat patients with dignity which, in turn, has a negative impact on treatment adherence.

Unavailability of anti-TB drugs is also associated with non-adherence to TB treatment. In 2013, India faced a massive anti-TB drug shortage. Almost every state across the nation had a limited supply of drugs like Rifampicin and Isoniazid, the first-line drugs used to treat TB. Paediatric drugs had run out and children were not being able to avail TB treatment in the public sector. Many were turned away from treatment centres. A study conducted in Mumbai reported that approximately 8 percent of TB patients missed treatment due to the non-availability of

---

32 Munro et al (2007). 'Patient Adherence to Tuberculosis Treatment: A Systematic Review of Qualitative Research.' PLoS Medicine. Vol 4, Issue 7. Available from: http://www.plosmedicine.org/article/info:doi/10.1371/journal.pmed.0040238

drugs.[33] The shortages, which can only be termed the biggest setback for the Indian government's fight against TB, reflect fundamental problems like poor government procurement systems, weak supply chains and inadequate methods of gauging demand.[34]

Then there are challenges specific to healthcare centres which deter TB patients from continuing treatment. These include: long waiting times, queues, lack of privacy and confidentiality, inconvenient times of appointment, poor maintenance of clinics and irregular attendance of healthcare workers and doctors.[35] The length of the treatment, the number of medications required, and fear of painful injections or drugs also 'tire patients out'.[36]

What Do Patients Need?

Treatment adherence is one of the most crucial aspects

---

33 Bagchi, Suparna et al, 'Determinants of Poor Adherence to Anti-tuberculosis Treatment in Mumbai, India,' *International Journal of Preventive Medicine,* vol 1, no. 4, page 231, 2010, http://ijpm.mui.ac.ir/index.php/ijpm/article/view/30

34 Anand, Shah and Mckay, 'Shortages of drugs threaten TB fight', *The Wall Street Journal*, 2013, http://online.wsj.com/article/SB10001424127887323469804578523262257381332.html

35 Munro et al (2007). 'Patient Adherence to Tuberculosis Treatment: A Systematic Review of Qualitative Research.' PLoS Medicine. Vol 4, Issue 7. Available from: http://www.plosmedicine.org/article/info:doi/10.1371/journal.pmed.0040238

36 Munro et al (2007). 'Patient Adherence to Tuberculosis Treatment: A Systematic Review of Qualitative Research.' PLoS Medicine. Vol 4, Issue 7. Available from: http://www.plosmedicine.org/article/info:doi/10.1371/journal.pmed.0040238

of curing TB. It is apparent that most default rates occur in the first line of treatment. This is because the patient starts to feel better after the initial few doses and quits treatment. In terms of the implications for drug resistance, this is catastrophic. Non-adherence to the prescribed treatment regimen has been linked with the emergence and evolution of drug-resistant forms of TB. For almost a decade now, the discovery of new-generation antibiotics has been trailing sluggishly behind in the race against DR TB. The emergence of an XXDR form of TB has made matters significantly worse.[37] There is an increased need to create strategies that ensure patients adhere to treatment and, in turn, manage TB in India effectively. These strategies include:

Universal access to quality TB treatment: The National Strategic Plan (2012–2017) promises early treatment stratification guided by DST results, as well as extending RNTCP services to patients treated in the private sector. The National Strategic Plan (2017–2025) promises to initiate and sustain all patients on appropriate anti-TB treatment wherever they seek care, as well as free TB drugs for all, universal daily regimen, rapid scaling-up of short-course regimens for drug-resistant TB and a DST-guided treatment approach. There is an urgent need to start implementing these documented policies.

Counselling and treatment education: This must:

- Provide information about the effects of medication to reduce the risk of patients becoming non-adherent when experiencing side effects;
- Stress the importance of adherence;

37 https://www.omicsonline.org/open-access/challenges-of-tuberculosis-treatment-with-dots-an-immune-impairmentperspective-2157-7013-1000223.php?aid=63513

- Sensitize the family, peers, and social networks of a TB patient about the disease, its symptoms, stigma and prevention; and
- Provide patients and their families a platform where they can access information regarding treatment, social benefit schemes and counselling services without being stigmatized.

Family DOTS: Families have a huge role to play when it comes to a TB patient's treatment, both in terms of completion and of carrying out an uninterrupted course. It is critical to sensitize and educate them. A family member can be tasked with reminding the patient to take the medicine daily, or with making sure that the patient doesn't stop the treatment after feeling better. Research shows that even when TB treatment was taken under direct supervision, the DOTS treatment being provided by family members played a pivotal role in a patient's complete recovery and cure.[38]

Economic support: Economic benefits are crucial for the TB patients who need them. They are needed to ensure that families don't live under crushing loads of debt and fall into poverty. They must also ensure that the basic requirements for successful treatment are met, such as the ability to buy nutritious food. In turn, treatment completion and complete recovery rates depend on economic stability. Such benefits must be extended to patients seeking care in the private sector as well.

---

38 Dave, Shah et al, 'Direct Observation of Treatment Provided by Family Member as Compared to Non-Family Member among children with new Tuberculosis: A Pragmatic, Non-Inferiority, Cluster-Randomised Trial in Gujarat, India', 2016. Available at: http://journals.plos.org/plosone/article?id=10.1371/journal.pone.0148488

Access to new drugs: Bedaquilin and Delaminid were introduced to address the emergence of tougher strains of TB such extensively drug resistant (XDR) and XXDR TB. Despite the spread of DR TB across India, the uptake of these two new drugs continues to remain slow. The drugs are stuck in a rigmarole of bureaucracy, costs and regulatory procedures. If India is to defeat TB as a whole, it needs to provide universal access to these two new drugs in both public and private sectors.

Forecasting mechanisms: A clear forecasting method is urgently needed to ensure the uninterrupted supply of TB drugs. A committee for forecasting must include representatives of the patient communities.

Partnerships with the private sector to harmonize treatment: There is an urgent need to engage with the private sector and design models of care with other actors, including NGOs and the government. Via a public–private partnership model, the private sector can play a pivotal role in scaling up treatment services, by implementing a strong referral system from the private to the public health sector.[39] The public health sector in turn should ensure that similar treatment regimens are followed across the private sector for effective management of TB in India. The following options can be explored by the public sector/NGOs in partnership with the private sector:

- Participation in referring, diagnosing and treating patients with TB;
- Establishing TB treatment centres within a private healthcare facility;

39 Uplekar, Mukund et al, 'Private Practitioners and Public Health: Weak Links in Tuberculosis Control,' *The Lancet*, vol 358, issue 9285, 2001, pp, 912-916, http://www.thelancet.com/journals/lancet/article/PIIS0140-6736(01)06076-7/fulltext?_eventId=login

- Conducting training and workshops with private laboratories and doctors to ensure best diagnosis and treatment practices are followed.[40]

Counting all who suffer: TB was declared a notifiable disease in early 2012. According to this policy, all private sector doctors are to notify the state authorities about any TB patient or suspected case. The idea behind this notification was to track the number of TB patients in the private sector. However, the implementation of the policy remains weak and India is unable to accurately report the prevalence of TB. For instance, according to a study published *The Lancet* in 2016, India missed out on a million of its population affected by TB in its official statistics. Under-reporting of the disease hampers health officials seeking to understand its prevalence. Reiterating and publicizing the significance of notification, coupled with strict action against those who do not conform, thereby emphasizing the mandatory nature of TB notification, will be beneficial.

Generate awareness of TB programmes: This may increase knowledge and improve attitudes towards TB treatment. Identifying and cultivating opinion leaders/peers in patient communities can help in treatment adherence and cure. Focused discussions on stigma are also crucial, since this is one of the major factors affecting treatment completion.

Introduce a patient-sensitive approach: Interactions between providers and patients must be facilitated. To this end, sensitizing frontline healthcare providers on the nuances of a TB patient's life may generate empathy.

40 Dewan, P. 'Improving Tuberculosis Control Through Public-Private Collaboration in India: Literature Review', *BMJ* 2006, 332, 574, http://www.bmj.com/content/332/7541/574

This can be done in the form of workshops, group discussions and trainings. The idea is to break down the mental barriers that people from all walks of life hold against TB patients.

A patient enabling approach: Concurrently, such an approach is needed to empower patients and enable them to have a part in the discussions and decisions around services and policy making—decentralizing the process in its true sense. Governments need to involve patients and their families when they decide about their lives.

Nutrition: One of the most important factors affecting the prognosis of the TB patient, the quality of nutrition directly affects immunity and overall health. We need to secure a mechanism in the public distribution system across the country to honour the Free Food Card for TB patients. It is of utmost importance for patients working in the informal sector and from lower socio-economic sections of society, as they have to bear the double burden of treatment costs and other opportunity costs, which both affect their ability to have nutritious food.

Transportation assistance: The public transport system should offer assistance to patients and caregivers for the duration of treatment and follow-ups, as the costs of travel act as a deterrent for the already financially burdened patient who has to make multiple visits to hospitals.

India is changing and it's changing fast. We need to take advantage of all advancements, such as the almost ubiquitous usage of mobile phones and internet, and harness them to provide better treatments, outcomes, adherence and education to MAKE INDIA TB FREE.

TB AND POVERTY: A MUTUAL RELATIONSHIP

Manasi Khade

My Story

My name is Manasi Khade. I am an XDR TB survivor. I come from a middle-class TB-affected family—my father was diagnosed with MDR TB. With two people suffering from TB in the family, the costs of testing, diagnoses and medication began piling up. Initially, we expected to be able to cope with the expenses for our treatments. However, we soon realized they added up to more than the family income. Eventually, we began borrowing money from relatives and family friends. TB impacted us not just physically, but also economically. We were extremely lucky to have such a supportive network of people around us.

Several socio-economic factors play a critical role in a TB patient's treatment seeking and completion behaviour. There exists an increased need to provide economic benefits to TB patients irrespective of where they seek their treatment from. The Government of India's recent announcement allocating Rs 500 per month to each TB patient in the public sector is a welcome move. However, we need to move with caution and ensure that the benefits actually reach those who need it the most. There needs to be an appropriate monitoring and evaluation plan to ensure that the benefits are being delivered and are helping the patients at the heart of the problem. At the end, we cannot address TB unless we address the poverty that precedes it and comes with it.

Poverty and TB in India

It is well established that the poor are the most vulnerable to health risks. TB affects a large number of India's poor due to social, economic and environmental factors; of these, poverty and undernutrition are the highest risk factors for TB in the country. Evidence shows that both these factors are directly linked to completing TB treatment and recovery.[41]

Poor nutrition is inextricably linked to poverty and hunger.[42] It delays recovery and also causes higher mortality among those affected by TB.[43] People with TB frequently experience severe economic barriers to healthcare, including high expenses related to diagnosis and treatment.

The other, and main, economic fallout of TB is the loss of income from days that one cannot work during this long illness. This is more so for people who are self-employed. The government's scheme to provide economic benefits while on treatment is a welcome step towards addressing this issue; however, since it is delayed, many will continue to suffer.

In India, new TB infections are not just the product of poverty, but also create poverty. Governments often

---

41 Nutritional Care and Support for Patients with Tuberculosis, World Health Organisation, 2013. Available at: http://www.who.int/tb/TBnutrition.pdf

42 The Impact of Poverty, Food Insecurity, and Poor Nutrition on Health and Well Being, Hunger and Health, Food Research and Action Centre (FRAC), December 2007. Available at: http://www.frac.org/wp-content/uploads/hunger-health-impact-poverty-food-insecurity-health-well-being.pdf

43 Oxlade and Murray, 'Tuberculosis and Poverty: Why are the Poor at Greater Risk in India?', PLoS One, 2012. Available at: http://journals.plos.org/plosone/article?id=10.1371/journal.pone.0047533

miss this underlying but strong relationship and attempt to address TB without addressing poverty. This is a fatal shortcoming as TB needs to be understood not just as a healthcare issue but a development issue.

What we need is to do is to fight TB and poverty together. We need to understand that TB continues to drain families and communities, pushing them into poverty. The economic and human impact of TB is many times greater on poor households and poor nations. The poorer the community, the more vulnerable it will be to TB, resulting in the possibility of increased transmission and infections.

The Challenges of TB and Poverty

Multiple challenges are faced by vulnerable sections of the population at each stage of the disease:

Delayed diagnosis: For the poor, there are economic and systemic barriers to prompt diagnosis, which may lead to continuing transmission. In the public sector, long waiting times deter people from seeking prompt diagnosis. The high costs of the private sector, which include inappropriate techniques for diagnosis and over-use of treatments that may not be needed, are major deterrents to correctly identifying TB.

Expensive: For most patients diagnosed in the private sector, the high costs are a deterrent to completing treatment. Research has shown that costs can lead to patients giving up on treatment. Alternatively, families often get into debt while trying to treat TB. Even when free medication is provided in the public sector, other expenses, including the cost of adequately nutritious food, combined with the loss of income, push families into debt and are disincentives to continuing treatment.

Loss of income: TB leads to economic and job losses and pushes families towards debt. In India, a study established that an individual diagnosed with TB lost an average of three months' worth of wages.[44] This loss in wages has a far more severe impact on those employed in the informal sector. Such a high toll often leads to interrupted treatment and forces individuals to give up. It can also lead to consequent mistreatment within families who feel the TB affected person is a burden, or outright neglect.

High risk of transmission: Delayed, interrupted and incomplete treatment due to poverty not only poses a serious risk to individual health, but also increases the disease risk to others in the household and beyond. Often, due to cramped living spaces and poor nutrition, others in the family also contract TB.

Poor nutrition and recovery: Poor nutrition among those infected with TB leads to wasting, poor recovery and often unsuccessful treatment outcomes. Nutrition is not just critical for recovery but also to ensure that a recovered individual can go back to living a fully functional life. The cost of providing this can also put an economic burden on individuals and families.

Mental and emotional health issues: Due to the constant demand for money, TB affected individuals experience severe mental and emotional trauma. Socially, people tend to avoid and ignore the patient and his/her family members, which can lead to depression and subsequent inability to complete the treatment. This makes the patient resistant to ongoing treatment.

---

44 Muniyandi et al, 'Costs to Patients with Tuberculosis Treated under DOTS Programme', 2005. Available at: http://medind.nic.in/ibr/t05/i4/ibrt05i4p188.pdf

Debt and TB: For poor households, the costs of TB lead to reduced consumption, sale of assets and greater debt, all of which result in further impoverishment. While specific evidence on TB-related debt is not significantly available, catastrophic health expenses are well established as the leading cause of poverty.

What Do Patients Need?

India cannot address its TB crisis until it makes concerted efforts to provide economic assistance along with diagnosing and treating TB amongst the economically vulnerable. From the patient perspective, some key ways to address the issue include:

Economic Assistance Programmes: Poor TB-affected individuals and families need **direct transfers of money,** paid as part of a social security system or a programme incentive. Further, transport reimbursements and treatment allowances paid directly to affected individuals are critical to ensure that they do not become desperately poor or fall into debt.

The Health Ministry's initiative of providing economic benefits to TB patients undergoing treatment as envisaged in the latest National Strategic Plan 2017–2025 is a progressive policy that is both patient-centric and compassionate. TB thrives in poverty and malnutrition, hence this scheme needs to be implemented urgently. To ensure maximum impact, it is critical that this scheme should have a clear implementation plan. Thus, it is important for the TB affected to know **when the first set of benefits will reach affected patients.** It's also critical that this programme is carefully monitored and evaluated from the patient perspective. Key metrics that must be considered include **ease of access, utility of benefit amount, exclusions and errors.** These are vital in understanding the impact of the scheme on patients. This scheme, if implemented early, would help ensure that, for the first time in decades, TB-affected families do not become poorer due to loss of livelihood or unmanageable health expenses.

Food and Nutrition Assistance: All individuals with active TB should receive a periodic assessment of their nutritional status and appropriate counselling based on their nutritional status, starting at diagnosis and continuing throughout the treatment. If unable to afford appropriate nutrition, they should be provided with locally available nutrient-rich or fortified *supplementary* foods to restore normal nutritional status. Food assistance improves access and adherence to treatment and mitigates the financial and social consequences of TB.

Community-based systems of care: Clinic-based treatment supervision poses a significant economic burden on patients. Also, poor geographical and financial access to health services often prevents or delays health seeking among people with TB. The creation or strengthening of community-based treatment supervision programmes would have the greatest potential impact on reducing TB-related costs.

Skill development: It's critical to consider what happens to TB survivors. It's important to ensure that they and their families do not fall into poverty due to lack of employment. In many cases they may be unable to continue with their previous work. Hence, training programmes or credits that help individuals or families affected by TB to generate income after treatment are very important. This is particularly relevant for those who work in the informal sector and lose employment due to TB. It ensures that families and individuals are able to rebuild their lives and do not fall into poverty due to TB.

While many of these suggestions may seem too difficult, it is important to consider that these are real issues that affect millions of Indians every year. India cannot call itself a developed nation until it addresses these issues comprehensively and helps its citizens fight a dangerous disease and also live dignified lives thereafter.

India cannot defeat TB until it recognizes and addresses TB as a leading cause of debt, poverty and financial desperation. For those with DR TB, the costs associated with treatment and diagnosis are significantly higher. It is time to think comprehensively and address the issues of TB and poverty together. Everything else, from the patient perspective, is insufficient and piecemeal.

STIGMA AND SURVIVAL: THE SILENCE AROUND TB

Keyuri Bhanushali

My Story

It was 2009 when I was diagnosed with one of India's most dreaded diseases—TB. For the longest time, I didn't want to talk about my fight with TB. I had begun considering it as my dead past. I didn't even want a mention of it in my future—only because, as a woman, I didn't want to lead a lonely life.

In November 2009, I started coughing and was declared allergic to sweets and fried food. While the prescribed medication did help to reduce the cough for a while, it returned with fever. This time, I was immediately referred to a specialist who diagnosed me with extra-pulmonary TB. The lymph nodes in my lungs had swollen up. I was informed that I will be put on medication and will be TB free in nine months.

However, even after ten months of medication, my condition didn't improve. In fact, a bulge was found on one of my chest walls. I was again referred to another private medical practitioner. It was he who finally diagnosed me with MDR TB. I was put on the correct treatment regimen and was finally declared TB free in 2011.

My journey with TB was fraught with negative thoughts. I always wondered: who would marry me? Who would marry my siblings? Should I talk about my TB at all or not? Why shouldn't I talk about? Is it because I am a woman?

How does stigma affect TB patients and families?

Most TB affected individuals or their families face stigma at some juncture. The common myths and misconceptions around TB are the root cause of this stigma. For instance, TB patients are considered to be cursed; it is believed to be an incurable disease; rumours abound that the drugs used for treating TB are ineffective, causing more harm than good.[45] Considering it's contagious, TB patients are very often ostracized by other people. This fear compels them to hide their symptoms and not pursue proper treatment.[46] It is shocking that people are still unaware of how TB spreads.[47] There is also an unspoken silence around the stigma which plays a pivotal role in creating this blanket of fear and sadness around TB.

TB is generally associated with poverty, poor nutrition and a lack of cleanliness. Hence, TB affected individuals and families are often blamed for having TB. Not all TB is contagious, yet the fear of infection leads to avoidance, discrimination and boycott. In the case of women, TB is associated with infertility, hence, in many communities, TB affected families or women from those families are not considered marriageable.

Why is TB Stigma Such a Challenge?

TB stigma is born out of ignorance and the fear of being

---

45 Stigma and Myths, TB Alert. Available at: https://www.tbalert.org/about-tb/global-tb-challenges/stigma-myths/

46 Cremers et al, 'Assessing the Consequences of Stigma for Tuberculosis Patients in Urban Zambia', 2015. Available at: http://journals.plos.org/plosone/article?id=10.1371/journal.pone.0119861

47 Myths about how TB spreads, TB Facts. Available at: https://www.tbfacts.org/get-spread-tb/

infected. It causes additional mental pain to patients fighting TB. Every person avoiding TB patients sends signals to them that they are inferior in some way. When they are isolated from their community, they feel as if they are contaminated from within. Such self-stigmatization in turn adversely impacts TB treatment, completion and recovery.

This stigma is not only the result of the disease but can also be the cause of it. Because of the prevailing stigma, those who are infected are hesitant to seek treatment. They ignore the symptoms for a longer period of time, thus worsening the problem.

The stigma also impacts one's mental health significantly. TB treatment is riddled with severe side effects. While these side effects may manifest differently in different people, they can cause immense agony and frustration. When this is coupled with the stigma many face, it can lead to severe psychological issues, such as depression.

Discrimination is rampant in workplaces, which may result in the loss of livelihood for TB patients. People infected with TB have to undergo all the problems of seeking and taking treatment while in hiding due to the possible affects of such stigma.

Finally, the stigma also impacts the ability to lead a normal and a healthy life after TB. Even after completing treatment, TB infected people are often unable to reintegrate into society.

Stigma is Gendered but Impacts Everyone

The gender disparities in TB epidemics are striking. While TB affects twice as many men as women,[48] the

48 Feng et al, 'Gender Differences in Treatment Outcomes of

brunt of the social stigma disproportionately impacts women. Misinformation about TB related to women's fertility is rampant, leading to greater and more severe stigma faced by women, ranging from neglect to complete isolation. Examples of female TB patients being divorced by husbands, unable to marry potential suitors, or mistreated by in-laws because of the disease are well documented.

Men are also not completely spared. The stigma of TB has rendered many men out of work—consequentially effecting other family members who are dependent on them. Men face ostracism, social abandonment and discrimination at workplaces as well.

Children too haven't been able to avoid the stigma. They are affected by their parents' illnesses. Sometimes, they need to drop out of school and take up jobs to supplement the family's income. If a child contracts TB himself or herself, then teachers and other students invariably make him/her feel unwanted. Taunting, sarcastic remarks and bullying are common.

Even healthcare workers don't spare TB patients. For instance, one of the members of Survivors Against TB was asked to stand outside the clinic, in the sun, just because she had TB. Once she was admitted, she was shifted from ward to ward as the nurses were not comfortable around a TB patient. Finally, her doctor had to intervene. This is just one story.

It is a well-documented fact that the quality of a patient–provider relationship is directly proportional to TB treatment intake and completion. However, how can TB patients expect care, if healthcare providers, their own

---

Tuberculosis Patients in Taiwan: A Prospective Observational Study,' Volume 18, Issue 9, 2012. Available at: http://www.sciencedirect.com/science/article/pii/S1198743X1461048X

families and society at large continue to neglect them due to the stigma associated with the disease?

India, which is home to the highest TB burden in the world, plans to eliminate the disease by 2025. Yet it doesn't clearly acknowledge TB stigma as a major impediment to this deadline. Why is this the case? Why do we as a society, collectively not fight the stigma of TB? There are several other diseases such as HIV and breast cancer, which aren't talked about in hushed tones anymore. What is so different about TB and its stigma that it cannot be addressed?

What Does India Need to Do to Make TB Stigma Outdated?

A sensitive and patient-centric approach, where care and dignity are given prominence in both the public and private sectors, is the urgent need of the hour. Conducting workshops to train frontline healthcare providers to be compassionate towards all patients is a necessity. Integrating stigma prevention as a core component of nursing and medical curricula will also yield positive results.

There is an urgent need to **sensitize and educate patients on their rights.** No one has the right to stigmatize or discriminate against any TB patient, whether they are family or community members, or healthcare providers. A TB patient must be made aware of this.

There needs to be a concerted effort to **create and implement strict workplace policies against any harassment** based on a TB diagnosis or the suspicion of a TB diagnosis. These policies must include a redressal system which can be used by an individual infected with TB, in case of harassment. In addition, companies need to create an environment conducive to supporting TB patients at offices.

Massive public information campaigns educating the public on TB and its infectiousness and non-infectiousness will play a huge role in dispelling the stigma around TB. Such large-scale campaigns must be substantiated by appointed brand ambassadors—such as respected figures, celebrities, or sportspeople. They will help the message hit home. As an example, the push for polio eradication roped in one of India's leading celebrities for a pan-India campaign giving culturally sensitive and scientifically sound messages about the polio vaccination effort.

The stigmatized individual often internalizes a sense of being at fault or tainted, as these are the values perpetuated by society. Such self-denigrating attitudes are detrimental to countering stigma and lead to a vicious circle, comprising low self-esteem, depression and mental agony. **Stigma-reduction campaigns** must be conducted to also address self-stigmatization. Further, **a gender-specific approach** to enable women to effectively fight the types of TB stigma that they face would be highly beneficial.

Studies to understand the prevalent notions, attitudes and knowledge about TB amongst communities are crucially needed. Solutions based on the findings of such studies would go a long way in addressing TB stigma. Such endeavours will also encourage TB survivors to be vocal about their disease status and enable other patients to learn from them.

If India aims to eliminate TB, it needs to work towards ending stigma by addressing its very core: the attitudes held by the majority. It is a long-term process, but with consistent efforts we can overcome TB and the stigma associated with it. Without eradicating this stigma, this pervasive and enduring disease has no foreseeable end.

COMMUNITIES AND COMMUNICATION

Deepti Chavan and Keyuri Bhanushali

Fighting against TB is not an easy feat. And like every major event in one's life, TB too leaves one with invaluable lessons. One of the most critical lessons for us was that, despite TB being such a widespread disease in India, we, like numerous others, had little or no information on it. As a result, there were delays in seeking care, which in turn perpetuated TB infection and fuelled drug resistance.

The TB paradigm is dominated by clinical and technical discourses. We have failed to recognize the fact that TB thrives within society at large. While the Revised National TB Control Programme (RNTCP) has now resorted to active case finding, it has largely been unable to engage with the community effectively. Other actors, such as civil society, which do have inroads into social communities, have barely been able to make an impact on community engagement. The media, too, has relegated TB to being 'a problem for doctors'. This makes the country as a whole, mute spectators in the fight against TB.

The Current Scenario

One of our failures in responding to TB has been communication. A cursory literature review makes it apparent that TB has long been a problem left to the medical communities and clinical establishments. TB has not been taken up as an area of communication within the general public. So, what is wrong?

General Public

There is **poor awareness and understanding** of TB overall. People exhibiting a persistent cough for over two weeks do not consider seeking treatment, dismissing it as normal. Those who are affected by TB, and their families, often do not know where to find help.[49] Further, awareness of extra-pulmonary TB (EP TB) is also limited. People are hardly aware of the difference between TB and EP TB. The idea of TB remains outside of popular discourse on development. Unlike HIV/AIDS, gender and other big issues, communities have not been informed or engaged about it.

The idea of TB carries with it deep-seated **stigma**. This is especially true in low- and middle-income countries. Studies show that in many cultures, TB is associated with pollution or weakness, or attributed to a curse.[50] People are reluctant to share their disease status with friends and family. There is rampant discrimination at workplaces and within communities. Those infected with TB often isolate themselves, viewing themselves as infectious. Eating together or sharing close quarters is

49 'Time of Action on TB Communication, A briefing for policy makers, programmers and health communicators on contemporary communication opportunities and challenges', Panos Policy Briefing, London, 2005. Available at: http://www.stoptb.org/assets/documents/countries/acsm/Action%20on%20TB%20Communications%20(PANOS).pdf

50 'Time of Action on TB Communication, A briefing for policy makers, programmers and health communicators on contemporary communication opportunities and challenges,' Panos Policy Briefing, London, 2005. Available at: http://www.stoptb.org/assets/documents/countries/acsm/Action%20on%20TB%20Communications%20(PANOS).pdf

often made uncomfortable or impossible through self-imposed or enforced isolation.[51]

Such stigma can also impact the process of seeking TB treatment and completion. Even doctors urge their patients to maintain a silence around their disease status, which only reinforces the stigma. Dual stigma and discrimination around TB associated with HIV/AIDS and TB/HIV co-infection is also emerging, with one feeding off the other.

Women, in particular, are disproportionately impacted by the stigma of TB. If a woman is of a marriageable age or is unmarried, her disease status is hidden, assuming that no good match will come her way. If she is married, then the challenges are enormous, given the patriarchal nature of our society. For instance, a married woman with TB may be vulnerable to abandonment by in-laws/husbands. If she returns to her natal home, the other people in the community talk against her. She is automatically isolated. This sorry state of affairs results in mental agony which is detrimental to TB treatment completion and cure.

These prevalent attitudes and behaviours enable the greater spread of the infection, which is quickly spiralling into an uncontrollable state. Lack of communication about stigma adds to the silence, allowing such discrimination to flourish unchecked.

Government

In India, due to lack of awareness, there is a long delay in between the onset of symptoms and diagnosis. Several studies suggest that on an average there is an estimated

51 Ibid

delay of two to six months in seeking the right diagnosis.[52] Such a long delay between the onset of symptoms and accurate diagnosis suggests a lack of awareness on where to find help. TB is highly contagious and infectious. An infected person can infect ten to fifteen other people every year.[53] The emergence of DR TB makes the situation even more disturbing.

While the public sector health system offers free TB diagnosis and treatment facilities, its consistently low TB detection and treatment rates suggest the lack of a critical element: communication to draw patients to health facilities. People in need are expected to simply come for treatment of their own accord, or to be referred by other parts of the health system. There is little active outreach to bring them in. The **lack of communication** is a key cause of this problem.[54]

Public-sector health workers play a crucial role in providing caring, non-discriminatory and quality health services to patients infected with TB. Their **attitudes and behaviours** have direct influences on the health-seeking behaviour of the patients. First-line caregivers have the most influence on the success of the TB control programme; however, relatively little is known about their depth of knowledge about TB control and the

---

52 Ibid

53 Media Centre, Tuberculosis, World Health Organisation, October 2017. Available at: http://www.who.int/mediacentre/factsheets/fs104/en/

54 'Time of Action on TB Communication, A briefing for policy makers, programmers and health communicators on contemporary communication opportunities and challenges', Panos Policy Briefing, London, 2005. Available at: http://www.stoptb.org/assets/documents/countries/acsm/Action%20on%20TB%20Communications%20(PANOS).pdf

extent to which health workers stigmatize TB patients. Insufficient knowledge and the high individual cost of treatment have been identified as the main obstacles to compliance among men, while sensitivity to interaction with health staff and stigmatization in society have been reported as the main obstacles among women.[55]

TB is often not treated completely and one of the most common reasons given for stopping treatment is **poor behaviour or mistakes by healthcare workers.** Many healthcare workers themselves consider TB patients to be unclean and link TB with AIDS, which leads to social stigmatization and discrimination. There is clear evidence of the effects of culturally influenced beliefs about and attitudes to TB, and their effect on adherence to treatment. Healthcare support as a facilitator and stigma as a barrier are diametrically opposed concepts; if healthcare workers perpetuate stigma, it shows the crying need for information on TB care and treatment.

Private sector

Due to the focus on **profit making,** a TB patient in the private sector is not given much time by any doctor. India's private sector is influenced by a stronghold of vested pharmaceutical and diagnostic chains' interests. The main agenda is to garner money, even if comes at the cost of human lives. The logical extension of this is that, in the race to earn a little more, doctors spend

55 Wou, Chou et al, 'Assessment of Changes in Knowledge and Stigmatization Following Tuberculosis Training Workshops in Taiwan'. Available at: https://ac.els-cdn.com/S0929664609600814/1-s2.0-S0929664609600814-main.pdf?_tid=06bc490e-1622-11e8-98fd-00000aacb360&acdnat=1519119783_cd988716e4577251fa666e7d2de23bc0

very little time on each patient, removing the opportunity for communication exchange. In the case of TB, such behaviour makes an impact on eventual treatment. It may also fuel stigma, impacting the patient's mental health.

Due to the **lack of communication in a patient–provider relationship,** important aspects of treatment, such as the role of nutrition and exercise, the importance of counselling and tips to deal with stigma, remain unaddressed.

Private-sector providers have so far remained **largely unlinked to national TB programmes** and the DOTS strategy for controlling TB. The large numbers of private healthcare providers represent a key constituency for health communicators.

Media

Communication as a tool has the tremendous potential of shaping public's opinion. If harnessed correctly, the media is capable of creating massive public awareness and aligning stakeholders, leading to a concerted and holistic effort in tackling TB. There seems to be **no action to bring TB to the public's consciousness** and onto the collective public agenda. This challenge is enormous, and can only be met through innovative and comprehensive communication strategies.

What is Needed?

Communication is essential to sensitizing and educating communities about TB. A targeted communication approach on issues of stigma and offering information about symptoms, diagnosis and treatment will go a long way in empowering communities, thereby tackling TB right at its heart. For TB communication to be a success, it is critical to develop and implement a multi-pronged approach that includes all stakeholders in India's TB landscape.

General Public

There is an urgent need to create and implement a multi-layered, multi-lingual community engagement campaign that includes information, education and communication (IEC). The campaign needs to be substantiated by interpersonal communication at a grassroots level. For instance, focused group discussions, identifying and cultivating opinion leaders from the community, and working closely with activist groups of TB patients can all potentially radicalize our approach to TB.

While the RNTCP distributes IEC material, its impact is limited due to the language, design, colours and images used. There is an increased need to focus on simple, clean designs with two key messages in each piece of IEC material. Publicizing the availability of free diagnosis and treatment in the public sector, indicating where to seek care and explaining the significance of counselling are some of the key messages needed in IEC materials. This will help people to find the correct health facility and also ensure that there is no delay in seeking the right diagnosis and treatment. Specifically:

Gender Focused Campaigns: There is an urgent need to conduct gender-specific communication campaigns to highlight the disproportionate impact of TB on women and non-binary genders.

Trainings and Workshops: Non-adherence seems to be related to treatment delivery failures. The health system needs strengthening, with intensified training and supervision for healthcare workers. Trainings and workshops to inculcate healthy attitudes and knowledge on TB should be prioritized. The public sector DOTS programme remains the best strategy to ensure adherence to treatment, as long as it is facilitated by education, holistic care, enablers and incentives. To enable patients to benefit from it, health education must be stepped up within the TB control programme. To this end, the psychosocial implications of TB should be given due consideration. Better communication between health professionals, particularly dispensers, and patients is essential for improving treatment adherence, even with DOTS.

Celebrity-led Campaigns: Asking celebrities impacted by TB to tell their stories can help raise awareness about TB among the general public. Work on HIV/AIDS and other development issues shows the importance of moving beyond merely building awareness to also promoting active engagement and local ownership of TB and its solutions. Similarly, other health communication lessons around the quality of public discourse, the importance of a cohesive social response and the importance of mobilizing from existing political platforms should be applied to the context of TB. Establishing existing baselines and setting specific and measurable goals to achieve a critical level of awareness about TB among the general population will go a long way towards developing appropriate communication interventions.

Engaging Members of Parliament (MPs): India's MPs have a huge role to play in the elevating the profile of TB in the country. Discussions within political parties and raising questions on funding or research and development plans in Parliament are examples of how MPs can contribute to the fight against TB.

Private Sector

Private sector engagement has never been this critical, as it remains the first point of care for over 70 percent of TB patients. Clear medical guidelines on cooperation with other state and non-state actors need to be defined and disseminated. A concise model of care for TB in collaboration with the government, civil society and the private sector needs to be developed and implemented immediately.

Civil Society

There is an increased need to build a critical mass of people who understand TB as a development issue. Too often within public discourse, TB is seen as a grim problem, largely to be avoided, and of little interest to the general population. Efforts to draw out the relationships between this public health issue and other elements of social and economic life can enhance the relevance and immediacy of the problem.

Patient-led Campaigns: Greater involvement of TB patients in all decision-making processes is essential to ensure better-tailored and more relevant policies. Spaces need to be made for patient-activist groups to participate and contribute meaningfully to the global TB control agenda, because at present they do not exist and tokenism abounds. When people affected by TB can participate in monitoring government policies, then a strong catalyst for change emerges.

Media

The media plays a key role by going beyond newsroom reporting that draws on dry statistics and official press releases. Initiatives are needed to embed TB within other spheres of daily life to help catalyze public interest in the issue and promote discussion. From investigative documentaries through to TV soaps and chat shows, a range of media formats can help place TB meaningfully into the contexts of popular discourse. TB communication must go beyond the usual flurry of media and communication activities around World TB Day—the only day of the year when there is any perceptible buzz around TB. Beyond the media, a range of institutions could be mobilized to embrace TB within their activities and agendas. Materials and tools could be adapted to help various groups, from sports clubs to faith organizations and youth groups, to do this.

Conclusion

The issues that should be addressed through improved communication are: the level of prioritization of TB control within health services, allocation of resources, accountability and responsiveness of service providers, participation by sectors outside TB control, community awareness (misconceptions, stigma and discrimination against those with TB) and community utilization of TB services. Community ownership and participation in diagnosing and treating TB are crucial to address the social, economic and behavioural determinants that affect heath-seeking behaviour, particularly among the poorest, most vulnerable and marginalized populations.

FUNDING: WHY INDIA MUST INVEST IN TRANSFORMING TB

Chapal Mehra

TB is one of India's severest health crises. It is an epidemic causing extensive human suffering and economic losses: TB kills close to 1,400 Indians every day and costs India more lives than all its wars with other nations (Pakistan and China) have, combined. Despite being curable, it has and will continue to cost India more lives than have been lost in terror attacks for over two decades. And in purely economic terms, it costs India close to Rs 15.6 lakh crores (US$ 24 billion) each year.[56] Clearly, the human suffering, loss of life, productivity and economic losses it engenders make TB one of India's significant challenges to being the developed nation it aspires to be.

India has recently announced its determination to eliminate TB by 2025—while TB suffers gravely from inadequate funding in the country. Although funding for TB has increased over the years, it is has not kept pace with the size of the problem. What's more, most of TB funding is absorbed in service delivery, which is problematic as there is little or no balance left for other much-needed activities.[57] The funding for prevention,

56 'Tuberculosis in India: Can we ensure a test, treatment and cure for all?' *Indian Journal of Medical Research*, Editorial, March 2014. Available at: http://journals.plos.org/plosone/article?id=10.1371/journal.pone.0148488

57 'TB India 2017', Revised National TB Control Programme,

public awareness and stigma reduction is virtually nil.

The Impact of TB

To understand the gravity of the TB crisis in India, India's policy makers must sufficiently understand its impact on Indians.

Studies suggest that on an average **3 to 4 months** of work time is lost for every person who experiences TB, resulting in the loss of an average potential earning of **20 to 30 percent** of the annual household income.[58] Hence, TB is an engine of death, poverty and impoverishment. It robs the country of human capital as well, afflicting primarily younger, productive adults thereby robbing generations of their capacity and potential. A 2008 study on the economic impact of TB control efforts estimated that on an average each TB case incurs a national economic burden of around **Rs 8 lakhs** (US$ 12,235) and a health burden of around **4.1 Disability Adjusted Life Years** (DALYs).[59] Similarly, a death from TB in India incurs an average burden of around **Rs 43 lakhs** (US$ 67,305) and around **21.3 DALYs.**[60]

Annual Status Report, Central TB Division, Ministry of Health and Family Welfare. Available at: https://tbcindia.gov.in/WriteReadData/TB%20India%202017.pdf

58 Muniyandi and Balasubramanium, 'Costs to Patients with Tuberculosis treated under DOTS Programme, Tuberculosis Research Centre, Chennai', 2005. Available at: http://medind.nic.in/ibr/t05/i4/ibrt05i4p188.pdf

59 Kumar et al, 'Seasonality of Tuberculosis in Delhi, India: A Time Series Analysis', *NCBI*, 2014. Available at: https://www.ncbi.nlm.nih.gov/pmc/articles/PMC3981520/

60 Ramanathan and Palanivel, 'Economic Benefits of DOTS Strategy to Patients with Tuberculosis after Implementation of RNTCP', vol 1, 2014. Available at: http://www.shanlaxjournals.in/pdf/ASH/V1N4/Ash_V1_N4_008.pdf

What Ails the War Against TB?

It's important to understand the unspoken gap between the idea of TB elimination and reality:

Lack of funding: India may have the will for TB elimination but its current approaches and more importantly, funding, remain inadequate to counter this disease crisis.[61] With every passing day, the decision makers are failing the people affected by the disease and creating further economic impoverishment by not making sufficient investment in countering the disease.

Efficiency and intention: The lack of appropriate funding and innovation creates a huge gap between intention and outcome. While, India's approaches are well-intentioned, in reality the full execution of even the existing TB control programme is grossly insufficient. This is due to funding delays, limited personnel and inability to address the supply side (services) in order to address the issues of the demand side (patient needs). The programmes need to be strengthened, expanded and made accountable.

Expansion to the private sector: Most Indians continue to seek care for TB in India's vast, unregulated and unengaged private sector, where care is highly variable and exploitation remains extremely high. This causes delays, high costs, incorrect diagnosis and poor quality treatment, apart from causing endless suffering to patients and feeding the epidemic. Expansion of TB care to the private sector is crucial in order to reach all TB patients.

---

61 TB India 2017, Revised National TB Control Programme, Annual Status Report, Central TB Division, Ministry of Health and Family Welfare. Available at: https://tbcindia.gov.in/WriteReadData/TB%20India%202017.pdf

Insufficient funding expansion: The proposed expansion in funding under the latest National Strategic Plan needs to continue. The NSP needs incremental funding increases which may not always be available. The prospect of funding increases under later governments remains uncertain. This affects the implementation of new approaches and strategies. Development and scaling-up of new strategies and tools is urgently needed to even remotely approach elimination. These will suffer from a lack of funding and as a result elimination will remain a slogan, not a strategy.

Key Challenges for TB Funding in India

TB continues to affect a large number of Indians, and funding gaps for the disease remain high. It is important to understand some of the key drivers of funding challenges:

Poor funding for health: Funding for health in general remains significantly low in India compared to the requirements of some of the health challenges. A small overall health funding envelope creates a zero-sum game, where one disease benefits at the cost of another. These challenges affect all diseases, but are especially difficult for those like TB where supplemental funding is needed to introduce new technologies and build public awareness.

Political will: India has recently announced its intention to eliminate TB, but this intention remains unsupported by the funding requisite to do so. Either political representatives are unable to grasp the gravity of the crisis and the amount of funding required to stem it, or do not see it as priority. In either case, across governments, there is insufficient political will. Funding has undoubtedly risen, but the increase is marginal, leaving numerous ideas for service enhancement unsupported. This indicates a clear lack of political will for funding for TB.

Low funds for innovation, infrastructure and research: The government seems focussed on delivery of medicines only, while controlling TB requires funding a new mission to develop infrastructure and support TB-focused clinical research. This is urgently needed, as the current tools and systemic capacity remain inadequate to address the growing number of DR TB cases.

Why Do We Need Greater Funding?

Some key reasons why India must invest more in TB control are:

High economic and social returns: Health expenses in India have been documented as the single biggest reason for pushing people below the poverty line. Not surprisingly, TB continues to be a leading cause of poverty, loss of life and livelihoods. India cannot be a developed power until it invests sufficiently in controlling TB . The disease disproportionately affects the poor and the vulnerable and is a cause of debt and discrimination within the community and the workplace. Investing in TB would help improve access to critical healthcare services, provide relevant economic and social support and help safeguard communities from debt and poverty. More importantly, it would help India realize its complete human potential.

The rise of DR TB: The increasing incidence of DR TB in urban pockets is a growing concern, as this disease type is difficult to treat and the treatment is extremely costly. If India's DR TB crisis continues, an enormous percentage of the current budget will have to be allocated to MDR TB diagnosis and treatment. As a result, other areas will be neglected. The best way to counteract it is to invest in TB now and stem the rise of DR TB. This is almost the equivalent of future insurance against rising health costs.

Disease control: Disease control is the responsibility of every government, particularly in countries with a large number of vulnerable citizens and communities. Early diagnosis and appropriate treatment for all (as suggested in the latest NSP) is key to controlling this epidemic. In India, this target remains distant. Current funding is insufficient for transforming the diagnosis landscape or for treating every TB affected Indian, as large numbers continue to seek care in the private sector. We need to provide free diagnosis and treatment for everyone. This will impact disease control and, in the long term, reduce India's TB related costs.

Neglect of other areas: Due to limited budgets, the focus on service delivery (of diagnosis and treatment) has always been key. This has led to other key areas such as prevention, communication and community mobilization being neglected. The answer to controlling TB may not lie with diagnosis and treatment alone but with empowering the public. The budgets allocated to these areas are rarely extensive and as a result they remain ignored. These areas however have a direct bearing on both disease control, early diagnosis and treatment. Increased investment in these areas is necessary to empower communities with information about symptoms and services and also reduce stigma—a significant deterrent for early diagnosis and complete treatment.

How Have We Benefitted from Investing in TB Control?

TB has been one of the high-return investment areas for India. Some key points:

- A total of 6.3 million patients have been treated under the RNTCP during 1997–2006. This has led to a total health benefit of 29.2 million DALYs gained, including a total of 1.3 million deaths averted.[62]
- In the absence of the existing TB control programme, the health burden of TB in India would have risen to around 14.4 million DALYs or have been 1.8 times higher in 2006.[63]
- The RNTCP has also led to a gain of over Rs 5.7 lakh crores (US$ 88.1 billion) in economic well-being over the period. In 2006, the gain in economic wellbeing was estimated at Rs 1.97 lakh crores (US$ 19.7 billion) per annum—equivalent to Rs 1,114 (US$ 17.1) per capita.[64]
- In terms of TB patients, each case treated under DOTS in India results in an average gain to patients of 4.6 DALYs and Rs 9,07,865 (US$ 13,935) in economic well-being.[65]

Conclusion

India must recognize that it is unlikely to develop in the way it wishes until it addresses its TB epidemic. This

62 TB India 2011, Revised National TB Control Programme, Annual Status Report, Central TB Division, Directorate General of Health Services, Ministry of Health and Family Welfare, Page 10, Chapter 2, 2011. Available at: http://planningcommission.gov.in/reports/genrep/health/RNTCP_2011.pdf

63 Ibid

64 Ibid

65 Ibid

disease is a significant obstacle to India's growth as a nation and to its people reaching their full potential. India must view TB not just as a health problem, but as a development challenge of its own—and include it in its strategy while addressing other development issues.

Most importantly, it must realize that with its current budget allocations, it cannot meet this development challenge of preventing TB and addressing patient needs. This will not be possible without an expanded funding envelope and political commitment to tackling TB. India must take the long-term view and evaluate the economic costs of investing in TB. It must also keep in mind the extensive human suffering, devastation, poverty and debt TB will continue to cause among its people if it does not provide sufficient investment to address this growing crisis. In the end, India will grow as TB diminishes.

LIFE AFTER TB

By Deepti Chavan and Saurabh Rane

Prior to our brushes with TB, we were on our respective career and personal trajectories. When TB hit us, it hit us hard. We were clueless and unprepared. We had no idea where to seek care from and how to even start grappling with the situation. Worst of all, our families were affected more than us.

Life after TB is not devoid of challenges. There is no guidance. There is a lot of confusion around complete recovery, relapse and care post-TB. But life after TB is as glorious as you want it to be. A question we are frequently asked is how does one rebuild life after surviving TB? Here are the lessons we have learned.

The two horrible years of undergoing intensive treatment because of our drug resistant status took our sanities and threatened to take our hearing, liver function and lives. We both lost part of our lungs to TB. We lost track of all the changes our bodies were undergoing. Even now, small everyday activities—walking, running, climbing stairs—are a challenge. We both still have issues with digestion, as the DR TB medication took a toll on our bodies. It impacted our ability to deal with the pain. However, we began taking small steps towards improving our physical beings. After a dialogue with our doctors, we both began observing daily exercise routines. A little bit of stretching and a balanced diet go a long way in nourishing one's body.

This is where post-treatment advice is critically important for survivors. They don't just need to recover. They need to **build strength**. The medical community, the state and the family all have a role to play here.

Apart from the exhaustion of shunting from one doctor and the next, the challenges of diagnosis, treatment and lack of information left us unhappy and drained. As if this wasn't enough, both of us felt our self-image going down the drain. Talking always helps, so talk about your TB. It will give you the confidence you need to remain afloat.

It's inevitable that TB will impact you mentally. However, recovering is a process that has to be worked on. You cannot let your life end there. Rather, allow the experience to nourish you with critical life lessons. We learnt ours. We were alone and subdued. It is critical to seek help. Engage with people around you—family, friends, your doctor—whoever you trust. Post-recovery counselling is critical in seeking closure and the ability to **rebuild yourself, mentally.**

Most importantly, believe in yourself; stay positive. Building a new life after TB is not difficult: all you need is faith in self. This, however, should be supported by the community and your family.

Create **social connectedness.** During our treatment periods, we felt as if we were never a part of society—for it was society which excluded us. Now that we have managed to defeat TB, we understand the importance of integrating our lives with a larger world. Of course, it is not easy. There will be people who may sever all ties with you, owing to your former TB status. But there are also people out there who will accept you whole heartedly.

Here, the role of the general community around you and the government becomes extremely important. It is vital to accept people who have survived TB. To make this the norm is only possible if large-scale public information campaigns are undertaken by the government to dispel any myths around the disease as well as the survivors of TB. For instance, many communities believe that TB is incurable and that chances of relapse are highest after recovery. This is not true. If one manages to develop and maintain a high immunity, TB cannot impact one's health further.

We have had to learn to **dream about the future again.** We feared forging loving relationships owing to our disease status. We feared that we will be rejected. But does that mean one gets disheartened? No. It's important to rather capitalize on the opportunities out there. You will have a full life to lead, after TB medication. The world is your oyster.

However, one needs to be self-driven. This is your road which you need to walk alone. Your family will support you, but this is indeed your battle, and yours alone. It is critical to find fulfilment in your personal lives. For instance, Deepti found a loving partner who married her and is a big supporter of her work as a TB advocate. One needs to keep oneself buoyant at all times.

When we finally managed to defeat TB, we decided to follow our respective careers. People told us how lucky we were to be alive... but that there was no point in building our careers again. We should not take risks and play it safe. We were appalled. Do TB survivors not have a right to professional growth? Are we to keep ourselves confined to our homes, just because people don't believe in our abilities? We decided to defy these notions. Today, we have not only managed to rebuild our careers, but are also helping other TB patients fight TB effectively.

It's been years since we recovered and yet every few days, we remind ourselves that we don't have to take those pills anymore; that we don't need to sleep upright tonight; that we don't have to be close to the toilet after taking the pills, anticipating that they will come out along with the rest of the contents of our stomachs. Yes, there is life after TB—as normal or abnormal you want it to be.

It feels like it was a different life. At times, we cannot believe that it happened to us. But then the scars from our surgeries remind us. They speak of a journey, one of loneliness, pain, tears and finally salvation. They speak of our road to recovery. Let's take a moment to just think of all those who did not make it: All those for whom life could not continue. The millions who lost their lives fighting DR TB. All those who are currently fighting DR TB and are losing the battle. All those who will not make it.

Trust us when we say that dying is easier. Defeating TB requires a tough fight. But this is not your battle alone. If TB is to be uprooted, then the government needs to play its part, the policy makers need to play their part, the drug developers need to play their part. Everyone that breathes needs to play their part because we are all at risk. We all play a vital role in this fight and we need to take action. More so, we need to demand action.

A significant challenge is the belief that the fight with TB is fought only in hospitals and clinics by doctors and other healthcare workers. While that is an arena where the battle is taking place, it is not the only one. This fight against TB needs to be fought by us all, not just the healthcare workers and the patients but the community at large. That is exactly what it is, a fight. Not just a personal fight, but a global one.

FUTURE DIRECTIONS: THE SURVIVORS' MANIFESTO

We have to begin by recognizing that healthcare, irrespective of whether provided by the government or private players, is a service with a clear end—the improvement of health and well-being. To this end, it is both socially but also ethically necessary to ensure that health services are easily accessible, affordable, appropriate and delivered with dignity.

In this section, we survivors have compiled the key recommendations from the focus areas of this volume as a final reference for policy makers, programme planners and other key stakeholders. Our goal in doing so is to create a final manifesto of key suggestions and demands that are urgently needed from the patient perspective. These are less detailed than the suggestions in each chapter, and point to more strategic activity needed urgently

While these may not be entirely comprehensive, they are representative and have been developed over extensive conversations, research and thought. We hope that the government and all key stakeholders will work to address these, to help all affected by TB to fight it effectively.

Drug Resistant TB

- *Count those who suffer*: A DR TB survey was announced by the government three years ago, but no numbers have been released till date. Continuous surveillance of TB cases and the building of a health management information system though data from molecular diagnostics is woefully absent. We need to understand truly how large the epidemic is to plan for the quantum of technologies and drugs we require to fight DR TB. **We need to count every DR TB case irrespective of where they seek care.**

- *Engage the private sector in DR TB care*: A large section of India seeks care for DR TB in the private sector. The government must create an effective partnership which ensures that every DR TB case is diagnosed and treated efficiently without unnecessary costs or delays. India cannot address its DR TB crisis until the government views this sector as a valued partner and its patients are given the same free diagnosis and treatment as those who access the public sector. **Everyone must have access to free and accurate diagnosis and treatment.**
- *Awareness and prevention*: We need large-scale awareness of drug resistance in providers and patients. This remains very poor and as a result DR TB is diagnosed late and often treated inappropriately. Recognizing TB symptoms early, creating awareness of TB among all populations and the medical community and renewing the focus on the fundamentals of disease prevention, nutrition, improved housing, income security and access to health services are crucial. **Every Indian should know and understand the dangers and symptoms of TB.**
- *Enhanced laboratory capacity and universal access to free TB testing*: India must provide every TB patient at diagnosis with a Drug Susceptibility Test, to rapidly identify MDR and more severe forms of DR TB. Despite the vast number of machines to diagnose DR TB, tests in India's public sector remain rationed. **Every Indian should have access to free, reliable diagnosis for DR TB as and when required.**

- *Ensure access to new drugs*: India must ensure access to high quality treatment for DR TB patients, including providing access to the two new drugs, Bedaqualine and Delamanid. This is particularly relevant for patients in the private sector. **No Indian should be denied new drugs irrespective of where they seek care.**

Private Sector Treatment of TB

- *Assured quality of care*: Irrespective of where individuals seek care, it is important that the government ensures enforcement and accountability so that healthcare is reliable and affordable. The RNTCP has developed formal guidelines to help local programmes structure collaborations with private healthcare providers and non-governmental organizations. The guidelines need to be enforced stringently. **Every citizen affected by TB should be assured appropriate diagnosis and treatment in the private sector.**
- *Seamless access*: The private sector can play a pivotal role in controlling TB in India, expanding medical outreach specifically in hard-to-reach parts, such as remote rural areas. This will also lead to increased case detection and notification of TB cases and the scaling-up of diagnostic and treatment services, if a a strong system of referrals from the private to the public sector is put in place. **In the end, every TB affected individual should have seamless access to care either through the public or private sectors.**
- *Free and affordable care*: Even today, most private sector patients do not have access to free diagnosis and treatment without enrolling in the government

DOTS programme. **Every patient must be able to access free diagnosis and treatment in the private sector.** This can be done easily by establishing partnerships with the private sector for:
  - o Participation in referring, diagnosing and treating patients with TB;
  - o Establishing TB treatment centres within a private healthcare facility;
  - o Conducting training and workshops with private laboratories.
- *Counselling*: **Every TB affected family must be provided appropriate counselling and information in their regional language by both the public and private sectors.** The government needs to establish protocols for this and ensure that every patient receives appropriate counselling through the government as well as the private sector, empowering them with sufficient information to deal with the disease and also providing the appropriate support systems to manage the disease.

Diagnosis

- *Free and accurate testing*: **India needs to provide a reliable and accurate TB test to any symptomatic.** Everyone deserves accurate, free and high quality diagnosis- whether in private or in public sector. There should be no discrimination based on where one seeks treatment and who your doctor is. Engaging with the private sector and providing clear medical guidelines and rationales for compulsory testing will go a long way in curbing the problem of inadequate TB treatment in the private sector.
- *Provide universal DST*: All doctors across India

must prescribe universal DST to all those diagnosed with TB. This will help in determining the drug resistant status of an individual and treatment can be offered accordingly. **Every Indian diagnosed with TB must have access to DST.**

- *Avoid shortages*: The government needs to strategically plan the stocks of TB testing equipment and cartridges. A clear forecasting mechanism needs to be put in place to ensure that TB patients in India do not suffer because of lack of drugs. **Shortages should be unacceptable in the public or private sectors.**
- *Introduce newer reliable tests*: Hasten the process of introducing new tests across India. There is a need to study and evaluate the performance of new diagnostic tests on the basis of feasibility, cost-effectiveness, reduced diagnostic delay, impact on clinical decision-making and patient benefit.
- *Research and development*: Focus on indigenous diagnostic solutions which are cost effective. Explore ways to combine existing and new diagnostics for timely and accurate diagnosis of various strains of TB. It is equally critical to monitor and evaluate each of these diagnostic techniques to ensure efficacy and accuracy. Regular assessment and quality control of diagnostic services and upgradation of equipment will ensure that the TB diagnostic industry remains well funded. **India must invest to make its own tests, suited to address its epidemic.**
- *Policy intervention*: There is a critical need to stringently implement the ban on serology-based tests for TB detection as well as to ban the use of IGRAs in the private sector for active TB diagnosis.

Treatment

- *Universal access to quality TB treatment*: The National Strategic Plan (2010–2017) promises early treatment stratification guided by DST results and to extend RNTCP services to patients treated in the private sector. The National Strategic Plan (2017–2025) declares it will initiate and sustain all patients on appropriate anti-TB treatment wherever they seek care, provide free TB drugs for all, implement a universal daily regimen, rapidly scale-up short-course regimens for drug-resistant TB and follow a DST-guided treatment approach. These documented policies need to be implemented on the ground immediately.
- *Counselling and treatment education is drastically needed in order to*:
    - Provide information about the effects of medication and thereby reduce the risk of patients becoming non-adherent when experiencing side effects;
    - Stress the crucial importance of adherence;
    - Sensitize the family, peers, and social networks of a TB patient about the disease, its symptoms, stigma and prevention.
- *Access to new drugs*: With the emergence of tougher strains such as XDR and XXDR TB, two new drugs were introduced—Bedaquilin and Delaminid. Despite the spread of DR TB, the uptake of these two new drugs continues to remain slow across India and needs to be brought up to speed.
- *Partner with the private sector to harmonize treatment*: There is an urgent need to engage with the private sector and design models of

care with other actors, including NGOs and the government.

- *Generating awareness* of the TB programme within the general public may increase knowledge and improve attitudes towards TB treatment. Identifying and cultivating opinion leaders/peers in patient communities can help in treatment adherence and cure. Focused discussions on stigma also enable greater treatment completion.
- Introduce a *patient sensitive approach* to facilitate interactions between providers and patients. Sensitizing frontline healthcare providers on the nuances of a TB patient's life may generate empathy. This can be done in the form of workshops, group discussions and trainings. The idea is to break the mental barriers held against TB and people affected by it.

Economic Assistance

- *Economic assistance programmes*: Poor TB affected individuals and families need **direct transfers of money**, paid as part of a social security system or a programme incentive. The Health Ministry's initiative of providing economic benefits to TB patients undergoing treatment as envisaged in the National Strategic Plan 2017–2025 is a progressive policy that is both patient-centric and compassionate.
- *Food and nutrtion assistance*: All individuals with active TB should receive a periodic assessment of their nutritional status, as well as appropriate counselling based on their nutritional status, starting at diagnosis and continuing throughout the treatment. If unable to afford appropriate

nutrition, they should be provided with locally available nutrient-rich or fortified supplementary foods, to restore normal nutritional status.

- *Community-based systems of care*: Clinic-based treatment supervision poses a significant economic burden on patients. Also, poor geographical and financial access to health services often prevents or delays health seeking among people with TB. The creation or strengthening of community-based treatment supervision programmes would have the greatest potential impact on reducing patients' TB-related costs.
- *Skill development*: It's critical to consider what happens to TB survivors. It's important to ensure that they and their families do not fall into poverty due to lack of employment. In many cases they may be unable to continue with their previous work. Hence, training programmes or credits that help individuals or families affected by TB to generate income after treatment are very important.

Stigma

- *Provide care with dignity*: A sensitive and patient-centric approach, where care and dignity are given prominence through the public and private sectors is the urgent need of the hour. Conducting workshops to train frontline healthcare providers to be compassionate towards all patients needs to be considered. Integrating stigma as a core component of nursing and medical curricula will yield positive results.
- *Educate patients about their rights*: There is an urgent need to sensitize and educate patients on their rights. Among families, communities

and healthcare settings, no one has the right to stigmatize or discriminate against any TB patient. A TB patient must be made aware of this.

- *Workplace policies*: There needs to be a concerted effort to create and implement strict workplace policies against discrimination based on any employee's diagnosis, perceived or real. The policies must include a redressal system which can be used by an individual infected with TB, in case of workplace harassment. Additionally, companies need to create a conducive environment to enable a strong support system at workplaces.
- *Roll out public information campaigns*: Massive public information campaigns educating the public about TB and its infectiousness and methods of transmission will play a huge role in dispelling stigma around the disease. Such large scale campaigns must be substantiated by appointed brand ambassadors.
- *Develop a better understanding*: There is also an increased need to undertake studies to understand the prevalent notions, attitudes and knowledge of stigma and TB amongst communities. Designing solutions based on the findings of these studies, to address stigma at its core, would go a long way in eradicating TB stigma.

Communities and Communication

- *General public*: There is an urgent need to create and implement a multi-layered, multi-language community engagement information, education and communication (IEC) campaign. The campaign needs to be substantiated by interpersonal communication at a grassroots level.

For instance, focused group discussions, identifying and cultivating opinion leaders from the community, as well as working closely with TB-patient activist groups, can potentially radicalize our approach to TB. While the RNTCP distributes IEC material, its impact is limited due to the language, overall layout, colours and images used. The focus should be on simple, clean designs with two key messages in each collateral. Publicizing free diagnosis and treatment in the public sector, where to seek care and the significance of counselling are some of the key messages which may be considered for IEC materials. This will help in attracting people to the correct health facility and avail treatment. It will also ensure that there is no delay in seeking the right diagnosis and treatment.

- o Patient Advocacy Campaign: Greater involvement of TB patients in all decision-making processes is essential to ensure better-tailored and more relevant policies. Spaces need to be made for patient-activist groups to participate and contribute meaningfully to the global TB control agenda, because at present they do not exist and tokenism abounds. When people affected by TB can participate in monitoring government policies, then a strong catalyst for change emerges.

- *Media*: The media plays a key role by going beyond newsroom reporting. Initiatives are needed that embed TB within all spheres of daily life to help catalyze public interest in the issue and promote discussion.

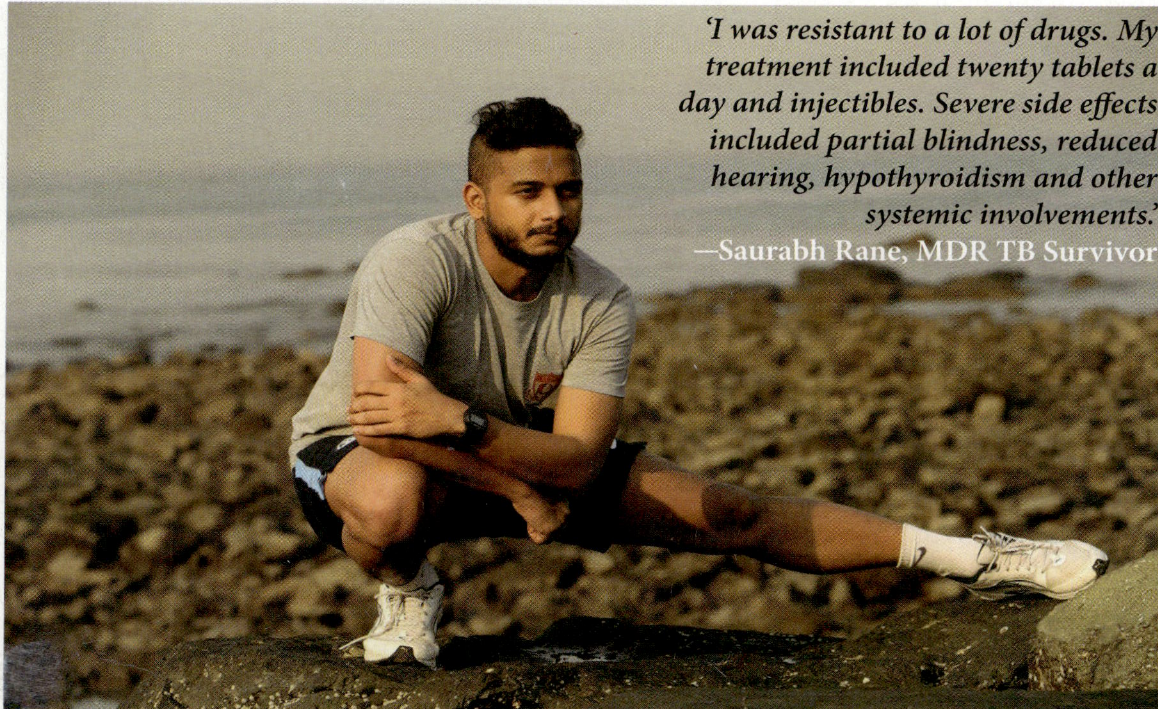
'I was resistant to a lot of drugs. My treatment included twenty tablets a day and injectibles. Severe side effects included partial blindness, reduced hearing, hypothyroidism and other systemic involvements.'
—Saurabh Rane, MDR TB Survivor

Photo credit: Prachi Gupta

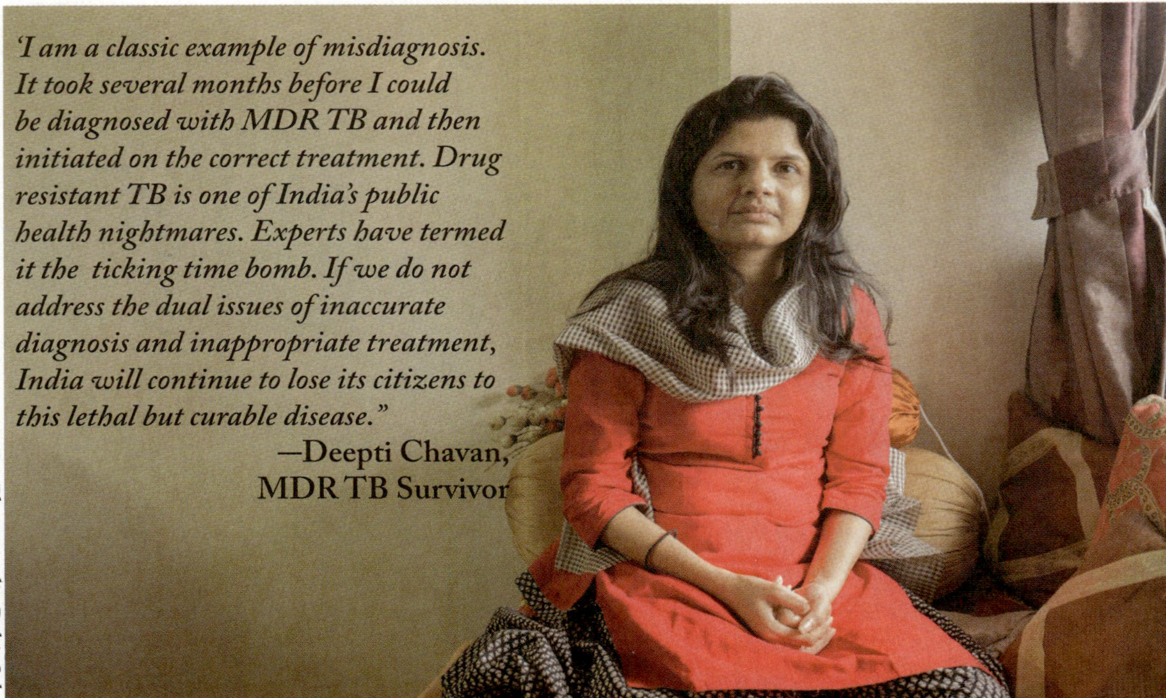

Photo credit: Rohit Saha

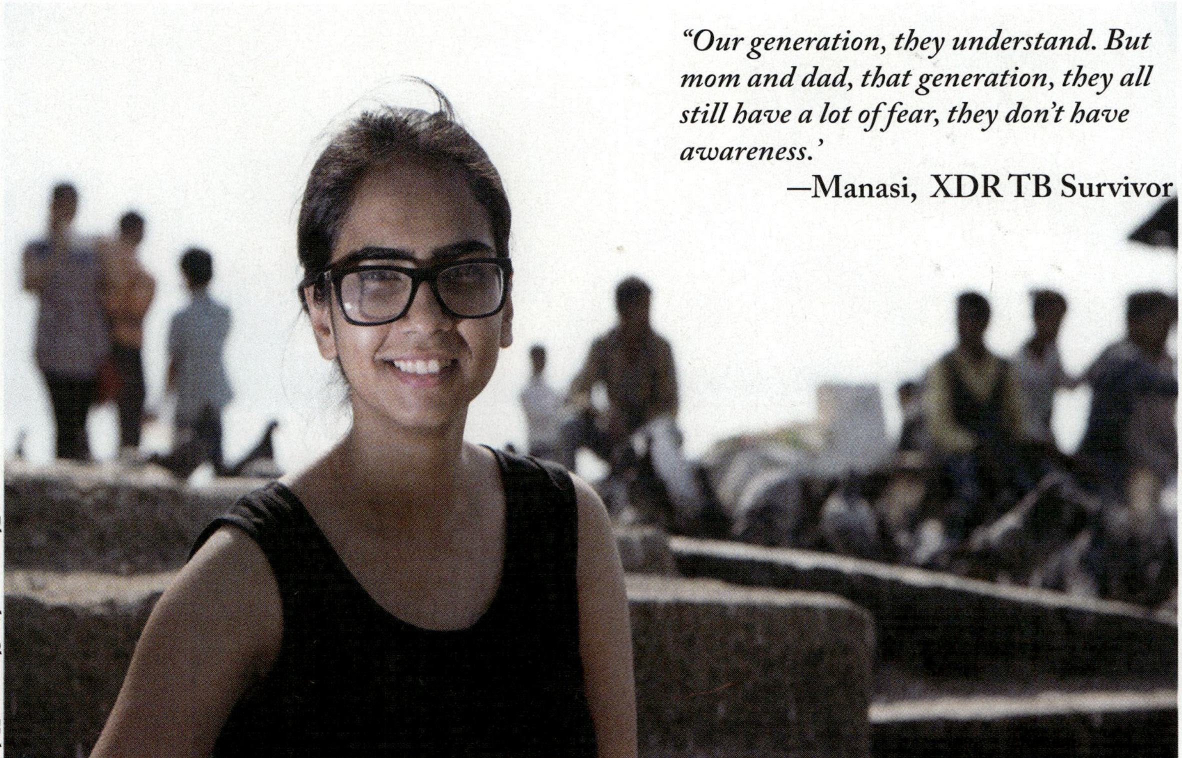

"Our generation, they understand. But mom and dad, that generation, they all still have a lot of fear, they don't have awareness.'

—Manasi, XDR TB Survivor

Photo credit: Shampa Kabi

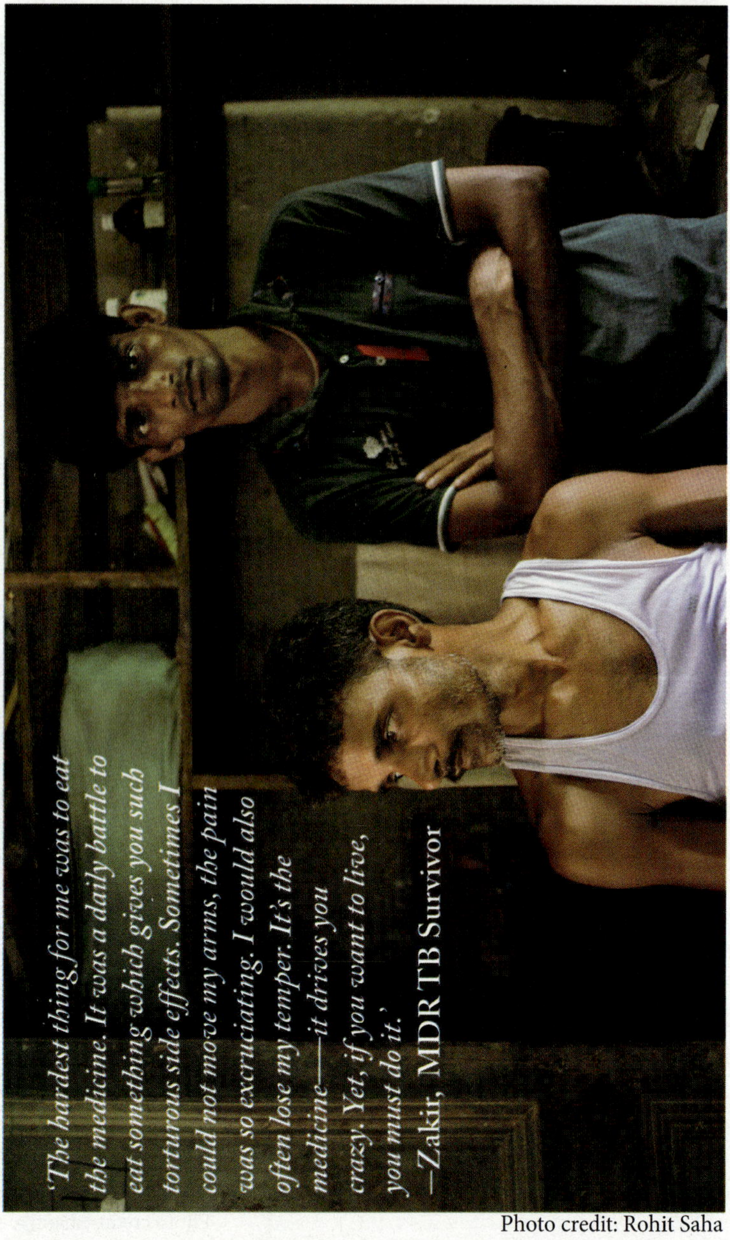
'The hardest thing for me was to eat
the medicine. It was a daily battle to
eat something which gives you such
torturous side effects. Sometimes I
could not move my arms, the pain
was so excruciating. I would also
often lose my temper. It's the
medicine—it drives you
crazy. Yet, if you want to live,
you must do it.'
—Zakir, MDR TB Survivor

Photo credit: Rohit Saha

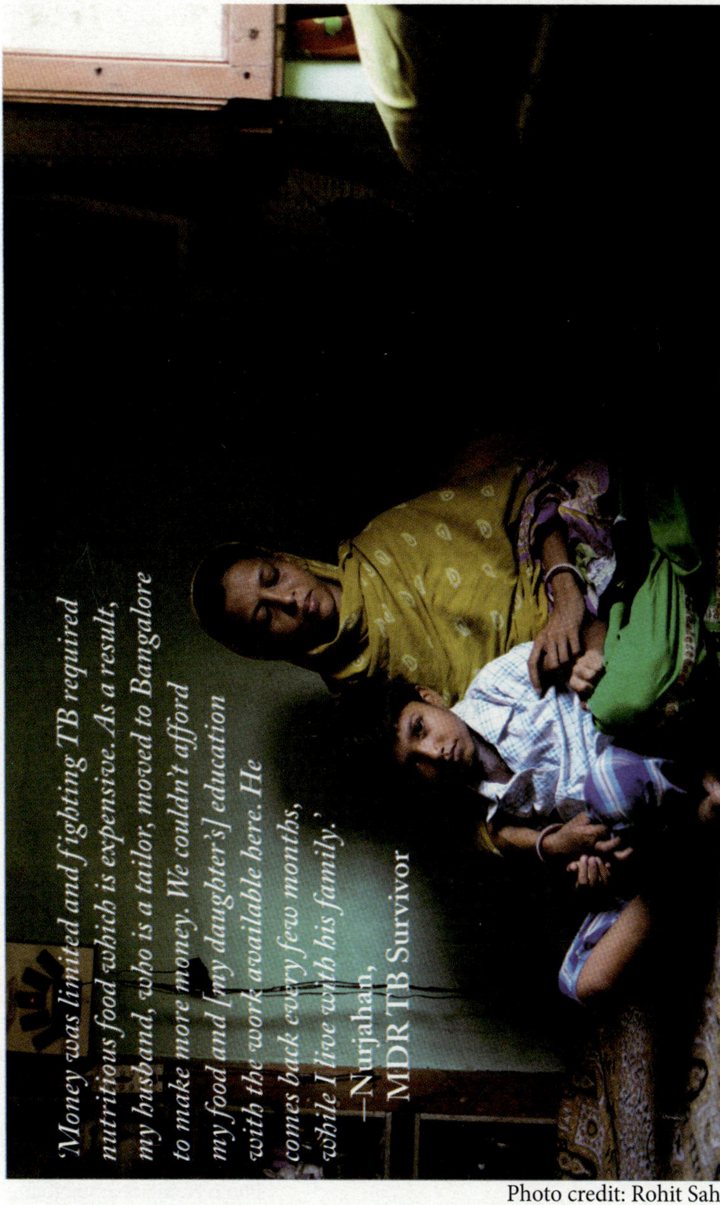

Photo credit: Rohit Saha

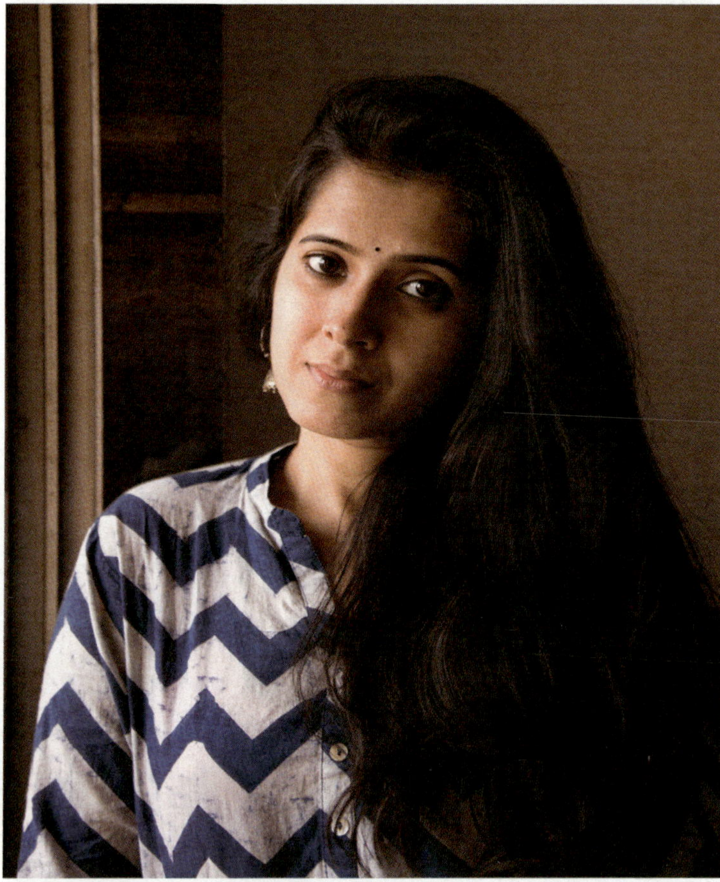

"'Who will marry me? Who will marry my sibling?'" These were my next worries. I, for the longest time, didn't want to share my story with anyone. I had begun to consider TB as my dead past. I didn't want even a mention of TB in my future—only because, as a woman, I didn't want to lead a lonely life.'

—Keyuri Bhanushali,
MDR TB Survivor

Photo credit: Shampa Kabi

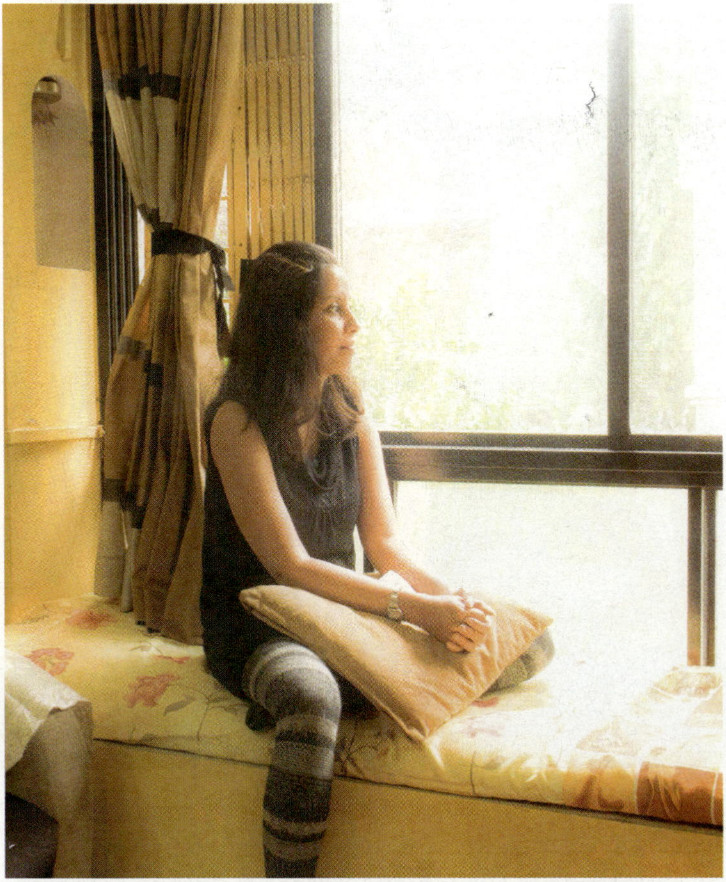

'When I developed a persistent cough and sudden extreme fever, the doctor prescribed some medicines, suspecting viral infection. He also asked for a chest x-ray. The x-ray gave no exact diagnosis, although the radiologist did make a prophetic statement: "You're going to be taking medicines for a long time!"'

—Debshree Lokhande,
XXDR TB Survivor

Photo credit: Rohit Saha

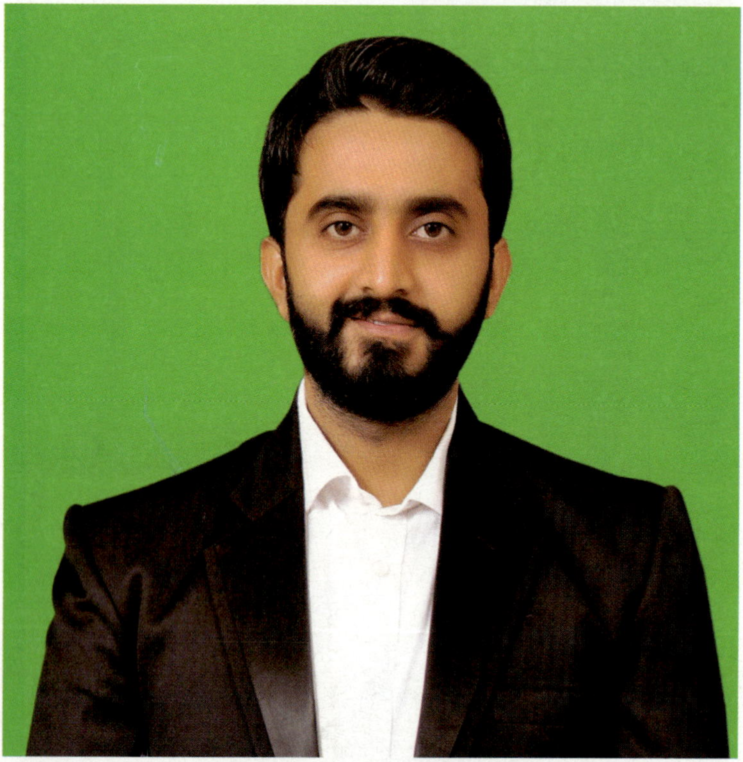

'After the intensive treatment of the first two months, my doctor wanted to change to a two-drug regimen. Given my background in public health, I was not convinced, and I discussed the new treatment guidelines for TB with my doctor. But he brushed me aside. I then downloaded the WHO-endorsed treatment regimen comprising three pills a day. I also called my friends in Central Division of TB (CTD) and confirmed that the TB treatment regimen was indeed being changed. Only then did I get the required treatment.'

—**Arun Singh, TB Survivor**

Photo credit: Arun Singh

ACKNOWLEDGEMENTS

Every participatory enterprise owes its success to people. This volume is no different. It would not have been possible without an incredible and committed team that worked behind the scenes to make it a success. These include Kritika Kamthan, from Survivors Against TB, and Shalini Krishan, from Speaking Tiger.

They worked with the editor and the survivors to document and refine the content to make it most suitable for the intended audiences. A special debt is owed to our reviewers: Dr Zarir Udwadia, Dr Sarmant Singh, Dr Puneet Dewan, Shibu Vijayan and Dr Prabhu Desai. Each of these experts guided this enterprise, giving relevant inputs and suggesting pertinent changes.

Finally, a deep gratitude to Dr Soumya Swaminathan who introduced this volume and has always been a champion of the survivor-led perspective. She wrote the introduction despite a grueling travel schedule and multiple engagements.

Each of these supporters have served as guides but also inspirations for this work.

ABOUT THE AUTHORS

Deepti Chavan is a MDR TB survivor, located in Mumbai. After undergoing TB treatment for six years due to misdiagnosis and inappropriate treatment, she is now married and a TB advocate and spokesperson for the rights of TB patients.

Saurabh Rane is a MDR TB survivor based in New Delhi. He is a doctor, who was infected with TB while completing his education. He took treatment for more than two years, while battling severe side effects. While still on treatment, he ran his first marathon. Saurabh is now a development professional, a TB advocate and a fitness enthusiast.

Keyuri Bhanushali is a MDR TB survivor who lives in Mumbai. Despite a series of misdiagnoses, Keyuri finally managed to defeat TB in 2011. She is an accountant turned copy-writer in a leading advertising agency.

Manasi Khade is an XDR TB survivor, located in Mumbai. She is currently a student at JJ College of Arts and is also a freelance photographer. She has documented other TB survivors and works with issues of health communication.

Debshree Lokhande is an XXDR TB survivor, living in Pune. Her battle with TB is a classic case of misdiagnosis and inappropriate treatment. Debshree is an architect by profession and a spokesperson for TB patients.

Arun Singh is a TB survivor, living in Delhi. He comes from a family affected by TB, having lost his father to the disease seven years ago. He is a public health professional.

Chapal Mehra is an independent advocate, public health specialist, and commentator based in New Delhi. A public service leadership scholar, he graduated from New York University and Delhi University. He has been working with survivors and affected communities, doctors and the government on issues of patient centric care, patient experiences, stigma, gender and disease. He writes extensively on quality of care, health system access, and human rights in health and is the author of two monographs *Nine Lives: TB and Women in India* and *Voices of TB*. He has written for *The Hindu*, *The British Medical Journal*, the Huffington Post and *Indian Express*. He is the founder of Survivors Against TB, an advocacy group working on TB, and continues to advocate on increasing resources for health, particularly TB and HIV, and addressing patient needs.